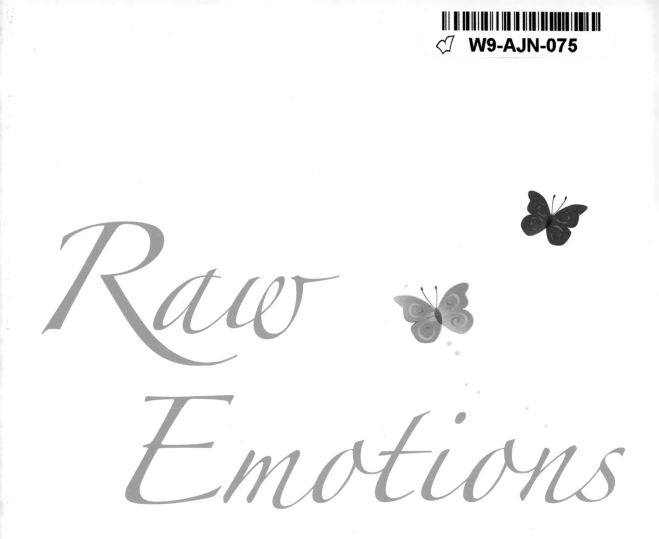

Raw Emotions

Angela Stokes

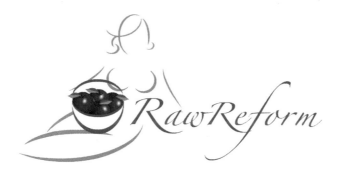

www.RawReform.com

the natural way to weight loss

Front cover artwork by Popowa Design. www.popowa.co.uk
Illustrations inside book by Desiree Martinez. www.desireemartinez.com
Selected photography by Petra Kuite www.petrakuite.com, Ellen Atkin www.ellenatkin.com and Terilynn Epperson www.thedailyrawcafe.com
Layout by Liz Johnson. jollyhill@gmail.com

Editorial and Design Inspiration: Susan Ure Reid. www.forthejoy.co.uk
Additional Editing: Kathy Glass. kathyg45@gmail.com

Library of Congress Catalog Card Number on file:
978-0-9795701-1-7

Printed in Canada

Praise for 'Raw Emotions'

I have read your new book *Raw Emotions*. I have to say that it is the best raw food book I have ever read so far – and I have read many :). You have done such an amazing job and I could totally relate to everything you have gone through. Very, very good job! Thank you so much!
--Sara

I've always wondered when someone would stop sweeping the issue of raw emotions under the carpet. In this tome of love, Angela gets deep down and squeaky clean! Her attention to detail, her consistent approach and her truly holistic guidance could cause you the revolution you've been begging for. Angela joins the dots with the psychology of happiness, addiction, cravings, emptiness and love. Her book paints a full picture of how you can become an ecstatic raw being. I'm so glad this book exists. There is a huge book-shaped hole on everyone's bookshelf that will now be filled with one of the most useful books ever on the subject of food.
Love and blissings to all,
--Shazzie, www.shazzie.com

THANK YOU for *Raw Emotions*! This couldn't have come at a better time for me as, despite embracing raw food wholeheartedly, I've been struggling with the emotional side of things after so many years of food having been my best friend/worst enemy. It has your characteristic warmth and intelligence on every page, and has so obviously been created with a lot of love. I'm reading it slowly so as to relish what is already proving to be such a great source of comfort and strength as I tread my path away from the darkness and into the light!
Congratulations and thank you!
--Kaye

Wow. This book is packed with WISDOM. There is no other raw book in the world that goes into such detail about the emotional journey that accompanies the raw path, as we learn to step into our truths and begin the process of fully embodying our divine selves. There is not a single page in this book where you will not uncover some nugget of inspiration on cultivating the emotional body in line with the physical body. This book is truly a precious shining jewel – just like Angela herself.
--Kate Magic, www.rawliving.eu

Raw Emotions should be out in Borders and everywhere in print form - it is the absolute best thing I have read on helping someone towards a raw mindset! It is beautiful, spiritual, practical, and I love it! Thank you! Worth so much more than I paid for it, a wealth of LIFE.
--Amy

Raw Emotions is definitely THE most thorough book I've ever encountered in tackling the psychological traps that keep people overweight and unhealthy. The great thing about the book is that I think a lot of it is totally universal in that the principles can be applied to understand and improve ANY less-than-optimal facet of life, not just our weight and overeating. For instance, I get how people can use it to overcome a lot of modern maladies such as: abuse, bad relationships, depression, procrastination, nihilism, etc. Other things I appreciate are the lovely, colourful layout and the warm tone of the book – it never feels judgemental, it feels like a friend.
--Anonymous

This book truly is a wealth of information. We are confident that any reader interested in really exploring, releasing, and finally overcoming their troubles with going and staying raw will obtain serious benefit with a read-through of Angela's *Raw Emotions.* She knows this journey, inside and out. She's lived it. She's been there, and because "success leaves clues", it's highly recommended that everyone who is considering (or has!) changed their diet significantly in the more raw direction, grab a copy and read with an open mind and heart.
--J&H Ohlander, RawFoodRightNow.com

You have just done a tremendous job synthesizing so much information, and I cannot tell you how grateful I am. Your book has brought together all the elements I need to think about and study and ACT on as an Active Transformer. You're an excellent writer (I'm an English teacher - it matters to me!) and very, very kind-hearted with us. Thank you so much for your time and effort with this book. It should be published for the widest possible audience. I truly think it's the best book I've ever read on recovering from food (and other) addictions. And I'm a voracious reader!
It moves me that a woman so much younger than me has healed herself so remarkably; your journey inspires me to make the most of the rest of mine. Thank you, thank you, thank you.
--Susan

I think this book should have the widest possible audience. It is simply superb: very well written and jam-packed with information on every page. So

many "self-help" books waste your time promising insights but string you along to a disappointingly limp conclusion. Stokes delivers from the get-go and keeps it up throughout the book with her keen insights, solid research and synthesis of ideas, and numerous helpful exercises. There is nothing silly, woo-woo or frivolous here - she respects her readers' intelligence and our ability to embrace real work to make real change. I felt respected and nurtured by this book and cannot say enough good about it. I'm a voracious reader and a fairly tough critic, and I believe this book deserves a huge audience.
Thanks again, Angela.
--RR

We all have issues, regardless of how they manifest themselves. And the fact that this information is coming not from a scientist crunching data in a lab, but from a living, breathing woman whose body is her showroom gives it credibility.
--Winston, GLiving.com

THANK YOU, THANK YOU, THANK YOU for writing this book.
You have hit so many nails on the head for me in this book, I am very grateful to you. I want so badly to heal my relationship with food and eating and you are such an inspiration to me.
Now I see clearly why my earlier attempts at being raw or succeeding with any other way of eating have not been sustainable. And, thanks to your book, I understand why eating raw foods can be an important part of the healing process. Maybe the time was right for me to get the message...and maybe it's about the teacher showing up when the student is ready. Thanks again.
Best,
--Arlene

Real and lasting life transformations rarely happen overnight but rather unfold like a flower, revealing each petal in due time. Angela gently leads those wishing to follow in her footsteps of healing and change in her thought provoking and powerful book *Raw Emotions*. Angela speaks from the heart with the wisdom and grace of one who has experienced the pain and shame of food addiction. *Raw Emotions* should be on every bookshelf, the information is that good.
--Rebecca Carlson, www.purelydelicious.net

Firstly, I appreciated the fact that you don't assume everyone with an eating disorder is obese, or even overweight. Many Western women have horrible self-destructive relationships with food, which manifest in many ways and can be as devastating as obesity in Western cultures.

Secondly, I love the way you never preach, but offer stories, suggestions and tips based on your own experience of recovering from a difficult relationship with food! It's very easy to be intimidated and put off by dogmatic, extreme approaches to eating, which I've certainly encountered in the world of raw food diets. I appreciate your "middle path" approach.

Thirdly, I really, really love your holistic approach – it's all too easy to assume that recovering from eating issues/disorders is exclusively about food. It certainly isn't! You've included so many simple, practical, creative, interesting and sometimes fun suggestions for approaching a healthier relationship with food!

Finally, I'm very grateful for your list of recommended reading. Thanks again for your work, Angela; I feel you devote a lot of time and energy to reaching out and supporting other people...and it's much appreciated.

Best Wishes,
--Jane

Angela Stokes is a catalyst for transformation and inspiration!! *Raw Emotions* is brilliant for anyone interested in healing physically, mentally and spiritually. Angela's words have given me insight into the reasons for my emotional eating in the past and inspired me in new ways to relate to myself and food. I felt deeply connected to her as she shares her own raw experiences and struggles. She is a light and everyone will benefit from her deep love that emanates from this book!
--Alexandra, www.mygoddesslife.com

I have recently read your *Raw Emotions book* and it is changing my life, thank you so much. The words in this book spoke to me on such a deep level that I feel profoundly changed as a person. There is much work for me still to do but I am confident for probably the first time in my life that I will conquer my food addiction. Thank you.
--Claire

Angela is a radiant and knowledgeable guide for anyone wishing to create a life of nutrient density. Her wisdom shines through in this book, showing us once again that exceptionally high levels of nutrient density can be experienced not just in our diets, but in our spiritual/emotional lives as well. Join Angela in her radiance and start by reading this book!
--David and Katrina Rainoshek, www.JuiceFeasting.com

Contents

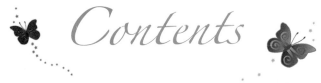

Acknowledgements

There are so many people I would love to thank for their input into both my personal transformation and the development of this book.

Firstly, to my dear Mr Monarch – thank you for all your support, understanding, loving encouragement, feedback and generosity of spirit. Your focus is exceptional and you help inspire me every day.

Many-fold thanks go to those who helped edit this book - including Simba, Margi and Joshua, Thubten, Kathy (thanks for dealing with my 'British–isms'!) and especially Susan Ure Reid, for specialist book blossoming services. Without Sue's extraordinary insights, loving honesty, perky reflections, pinpoint attention to detail and way with words, this book would have grown into a very different flower than it is today. THANK YOU so much. Your many suggestions truly helped shape this text into a powerful offering, which is now helping to empower so many other people - much, much gratitude to you.

A lotus blossom of appreciation too, to the five raw goddesses who helped illustrate and lay out this book: Sara for the cover, Desiree for the illustrations inside the book, Petra and Terilynn for photography and Liz for the masterful layout. You have all brought the text to life so beautifully - thank you.

To dear friends who have helped co-create and enjoy this journey along the way: Lara, Kate, Michelle, Caro, Zoe, Happy, Laine, Lisa, Laura, Shazzie, Kathy, Victoria, Deej, Paul, Justin, Mark and many dear friends in Iceland, including Heiða, Katrín, Magga, Bjargey, Inga Hanna, Þórunn, Þurí, María, Solla, Gíslí and Ýmir. Thank you *all* for the inspiration, love and hugs. Abundant gratitude also goes to the fellowship of Overeaters Anonymous and other '12 Step' groups, for holding a healing space that allows recovery to unfold. There are of course *countless* other people who have touched my life and inspired me in some way - I hope you know who you are (in every sense!) and that you're enjoying the journey...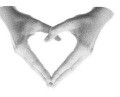

To dearest Jeanette, deep and sincere thanks for all that you have shared with me. Your generosity, truth and positivity have been wondrous gifts. Thank you for telling me what you see in me, for genuine mirroring and wonderful encouragement.

To beautiful goddess Anastasia, thank you so much si*star*, for the glorious visions and inspiration – we breathe deeply with you.

Thanks to my blood family, especially to my parents, without whose **support** for my education and sense of adventure, I would not have experienced the fullness of life that helped shape the person I am today.

Thanks as always to Spirit for guiding me.

Last, yet by no means least, thanks, love and appreciation to all those who've supported my sharing of this healing message since the start of the RawReform website in 2004. Thanks to all the readers for the lovely feedback, letting me know what the site means to you and keeping me updated on your individual progress stories. It's a heart-warming experience.

Best wishes, blessings and love to all, always, in all ways,
Angela. xxx

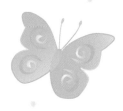

Foreword by Victoria Boutenko

Being a brave woman and an authentic writer, Angela Stokes has created a book that will affect all who read it. First Angela healed herself, and now she is helping others to overcome one of the most common and difficult conditions - obesity. There are very few people in the world who are able to lose 160 pounds using a natural lifestyle.
I consider these people to be heroes, because they are pioneers who lay the way for many others to follow. Angela is such a hero. I am deeply touched by her authenticity, her willingness to share her personal struggle without pretension. When I read her book, I could relate to many of the author's personal memories and anecdotes. By being sincere to the point of vulnerability, Angela is able to make a strong, intimate connection to the reader.

Having lived as a morbidly obese person for a number of years, Angela knows firsthand what it takes to be in the public eye day after day, trying and failing, and at times feeling hopeless. Out of compassion for all people, and especially the obese, Angela took the time to do the necessary research, describe her own success, and create a technique that would enable others to heal themselves.

Raw Emotions offers readers a thorough insight into little-researched fields such as emotional relationships with food, overcoming cravings, motives for overeating, and 'emotional detox'. This book contains many helpful techniques for handling cravings, and transforming obsessive-compulsive patterns into self-empowering habits. Angela is enthusiastic about everyone's ability to move forward toward their own optimal vision of how they would love to live. *Raw Emotions* could serve both as a guidebook and as a catalyst for major shifts, helping readers to discover a profound new potential in themselves.

Victoria Boutenko
Raw Food Author and Speaker
www.RawFamily.com
Ashland, Oregon
Sept. 2008

Author's Foreword

I'm very excited to finally be sharing my thoughts about the 'deeper' elements of healing, beyond the physical changes, which can unfold with a raw food lifestyle. This book has been a long time coming for me. It is the culmination of a great deal of research and experience during my own recovery, on every level of my being, as well as observations of those I coach.

I see so many people living with illnesses like obesity, diabetes, degenerative diseases and so on, feeling miserable and with no apparent sense of connection or genuine purpose in this world. So many seem knitted in to highly destructive patterns of eating foods that undermine both their physical health and total well-being, none of which is truly necessary.

How do I know that there are healthy, natural ways to reverse situations like these?

I am *living* proof!

Just seven years ago, I weighed nearly 300 pounds (21 stone/133 kg) and was miserable, anxious, resentful and lonely. Since starting my raw food journey, my life has turned inside-out and is virtually unrecognisable from the one I knew before.
I am now genuinely happy, healthy and feel connected to all of life around me, on a joyous path of learning and loving. Raw food was my avenue into healing on all levels of my being.

My 'Amazing Transformation' story has been widely publicised in the press and media. Most often, it is my stunning weight loss (more than 160 pounds released) that impresses and inspires people. Yet raw food transformation offers so much more than this. Shifts can unfold on levels of your being that you might not even have had much sense of before. Sometimes the road can feel a little rocky, as our bodies let go of energies we have been holding in our cells for a long time. I've been there, and I'm coming up smiling. This book contains concepts and tips that have helped *me*,

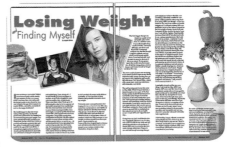

so perhaps they can also help guide *you* in *your* emotional and spiritual healing, alongside your physical transformation.

Living as a raw foodist, the common addicted relationship with food can change dramatically, as you're no longer taking in toxic, processed foods that are physiologically addictive and cause the most damage - thus, half the 'battle' is already won. Changing *what* you eat makes a great deal of difference. *However*, I've found that the emotional/mental/spiritual aspects of transformation often require much more attention than a simple change in food choices. The eating patterns we have established with food over many years – for comfort, excitement, reward and so on – do not simply vanish overnight, just by going raw.

Raw Emotions follows on from where my earlier books left off. Those focus much more on the *physical* aspects of a raw lifestyle. So, if you are new to raw foods and/or unfamiliar with my work, you may find it helpful to read those books first. (You can purchase them at http://store.RawReform.com.) For practical guidance about what/when/how/why to eat raw, see my first book *How to Go Raw for Weight Loss*. My next book *Revealing the Physical Changes* goes into detail about the physical effects we can expect in the body when we go raw, such as detox, colon changes, skin/body care and so on.

This book, *Raw Emotions*, is a work of love, in every sense. In my experience, a book does not simply get written out, sentence by sentence and page by page until completion. (I have far too much Virgo in my chart for that to happen!) The finished product, like any substantial project, seems to belie its own construction. Putting it together is like assembling a jigsaw with many thousands of pieces, jiggling each one gradually into place, all within the daily rhythms of life. A book gets written amidst juicing sessions, workouts, conversations, meals, interjections, sleeping and socialising. The focus required to polish the content and prose at times feels so intense that one wonders if the piece will ever be complete. Yet now it's here after quite a birthing process. May you find inspiration within these pages and enjoy your own smooth and sublime healing journey...

All blessings,
Angela. xxx

P.S. A little word of warning: I'm originally from England and I tend towards

British spellings and grammar, which can sometimes confuse readers in North America. So if you find an 's', for example, where you might expect a 'z' – e.g. 'realise' rather than 'realize' – please understand that this is the British convention, not a consistent typo! Similarly you might notice spellings such as 'colour' rather than 'color' and differences in grammar such as single quotation marks rather than double and so on. I trust these differences will only add an extra element of adventure for you as you read, rather than detract from your experience. Enjoy!

Introduction

My hope is that this book will help empower you to take responsibility for your own health and well-being. This is not a 'MUST DO', rather a 'CAN DO' book. If you don't already, I hope you come to realise and accept that *you have all the power you need* within you to make positive choices that serve you. You do not need anyone else – including me – to make those choices for you or to feel okay in your life. I am not here to tell you what is 'right' or 'wrong' or to give you a list of things you *must* do to be acceptable. I do not believe that would feel truly liberating or empowering for you. I *am* here to offer guidance and give you an idea of what's available in the way of support. You are free at all times to make your *own* choices, based on what feels good and resonates for you.

Raw Emotions weaves together the ideas of a raw food lifestyle with spiritual practices, emotional release work and self-help methods. Some people seem to attach a certain stigma to the idea of 'self-help/self-development'. As I see things, this path is about taking responsibility for *ourselves* – ceasing to give our power away to anyone, whether doctors, psychiatrists, partners or friends. We can become living expressions of our authentic selves, by ourselves – no doctors or medications needed. Self-help/self-development tools are suggestions, therefore, to help us on this journey, as we release habits that no longer serve our optimal well-being and instead try out and adopt new, supportive habits that truly nurture us. After all, if we're not willing to seek healing and a new path for *ourselves*, it's unlikely that anyone else is going to bring that to us. We are each free to step into our own glorious power.

> *"I would not interfere with any creed of yours,*
> *or want to appear that I have all the cures.*
> *There is so much to know...*
> *So many things are true...*
> *The way my feet must go may not be best for you.*
> *And so, I give this spark of what is light to me,*
> *to guide you through the dark,*
> *but not tell you what to see."*
> *--Author Unknown*

Many people who start on the raw food path don't realise the full potential for transformation that they are awakening in themselves. Sometimes there is even the sense that being raw is 'cool' or 'hip', while the reality that this is usually a **profound** and intensely healing journey is overlooked.

For most people, switching to raw means the start of a markedly different way of life and if we're not prepared for that, it can come as a big shock. So, it's wise to get support and take things slowly at first, especially if those close to you are not joining you on this path. Without support and a gently measured pace, it can feel like a dramatic shift for all involved and you might find yourself swiftly falling 'off the wagon' with a bump.

I often see a certain pattern at raw food retreats. People arrive with the idea that they might lose a few pounds, learn a few recipes and so on. They do not yet have a notion of the *extent* of transformation that may be in store for them, beyond the physical. I find it absolutely beautiful to see how they metamorphose in the healing space of a retreat and later emerge as radiant raw beings, transformed on so many levels beyond a few shifted pounds.

However, not everyone embarks on a raw food journey in the secure space of an organised retreat. Many, in fact, can feel isolated, confused and unprepared, especially when issues rise up in them to be released. For example, they may eat mainly raw for a few months and feel they have a handle on what to eat, then suddenly feel overwhelmed by all the emotions that are bubbling up for them. They might wonder 'where is all this emotional stuff coming from...?' and even question if the raw lifestyle suits them, as they feel so 'wobbly'. That's where this book comes in. You can think of *Raw Emotions* as your loyal companion on your incredible healing journey. It is your guide, here to help you stay on course; your own daily 'mini-retreat' that supports *your* radiant raw transformation, beyond the physical...

In *Raw Emotions* we begin with an overview of how we might have been re-
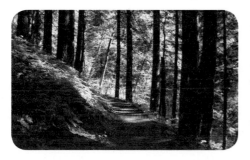
lating to food so far in life, especially in terms of our emotional dynamics and any addictive eating patterns. As you read about the seven different ways we seem to interact with food, you might start to see where *you* fit into the picture. We explore the nature of addictions and cravings - what ours might be like and how it is to live with them.

In the next section 'Where Would You Like To Go?', we focus on moving *beyond* addictions and limiting beliefs. You'll be creating your Optimal Vision for how you would LOVE to live your life. This leads us into a chapter on healing our emotional relationship with food and finding balance. You will learn about the three key steps I guide people through to help relinquish other-than-optimal foods and habits. We then consider from a broader perspective what it's like to go through emotional detoxification and what we might be looking to release, *beyond* the food.

In the main 'Guidance' section, we come to the true core of this book, where we can fill our 'Treasure Boxes' with useful tips, tools and ideas for a more vibrant, joyous life connection. You'll find a bumper collection of sixty key suggestions here: twenty 'Recovery Concepts' and forty 'Healthy Action Tips'. All are offered to help brighten your life and nurture a deeper sense of connection.

In the final sections you'll find a recommended reading list and tips to help you maintain a happy balance in your life, plus a Transformation Checklist for future reference.
There are also three appendices:

*Appendix A contains twenty tips for eating healthily as a raw foodist.
*Appendix B gives you ten simple raw recipes.
*Appendix C, a handy Resources Guide, shows you where to find services and products mentioned in the text.

You may find some of the concepts we'll be looking at in this book slightly or well beyond the realms of what seems comfortable or familiar to you. To get the most out of *Raw Emotions*, it helps to suspend disbelief and reactionary judgement while reading and to remain open.

Take a look at the health of the majority of people around you. Are they glowing with vitality? Or are they miserable, dealing with obesity, heart disease, diabetes, cancer and other ailments? Could it be possible that most of what you've learned about nutrition so far was other-than-optimal and doesn't really serve your greatest health? Perhaps there is some important information you simply never knew. Could it be that there's a deeper truth and another way of living that might bring you greater health and more joy?

By now, you'll know that I believe there is. In fact, I don't just believe it, I *know*. I am *living proof*. So I hope you'll allow yourself to stay open while reading, to the possibility that there's another way.

A raw foods lifestyle is an entirely natural way of healing that cleanses the physical body while also encouraging us to refresh our emotional and spiritual well-being. (Not to mention improved mental health, finances, relationships and more...)

Many of us routinely eat to the point of feeling 'stuffed', because we're looking for some feeling of satiation and yet overeating like this is not at all beneficial for our well–being – the body does not need all that extra food. In this book you can discover many other ways to 'fill yourself up' and feel satisfied beyond eating food, such as sharing quality time and love with others. You can learn to lovingly release unsupportive patterns like this and restructure your relationship with food.

When I write about 'recovery', I'm referring to reclaiming a happy, simple, joyous connection with nature and all of life. I'm referring to a life where you feel consistently great, eat nourishing foods in appropriate amounts and enjoy vibrant health and well-being. I'm encouraging recovery from toxic processed foods, disjointed emotions and empty life paths, into a feeling of radiance, joy and balance. This, to me, is the power of raw recovery.

You may not resonate with *all* that is written here – that's fine – please just remember, here as elsewhere, to take in what serves you and leave the rest.

Eating/Feeling Patterns

Just as most of us were not brought up with a raw food lifestyle (which we may now consider optimal), few of us seem to have been encouraged to *emotionally* express ourselves optimally either, as we were growing up. Rather than *expressing* our true feelings vocally or otherwise, we often learn to use food as a coping mechanism, 'eating over' our stress and *sedating* our feelings instead. As raw food speaker Roz Gruben so accurately pinpoints in her talks, it's challenging to process strong emotions *and* digest food at the same time. So, by eating at times of stress, we can literally 'numb' ourselves out emotionally. By adopting such habits, many of us have created strong **emotional patterns** around food. A powerful psychological component in our food choices is typically eating for 'comfort'.

What do we mean by 'patterns'? Patterns might be anything in our lives that we habitually/repeatedly do: customary ways in which we behave, things we tend to experience again and again, our typical emotional responses and so on. This could be *anything*, from always buying a certain type of bread from a certain baker, to never having quite enough money to pay for the things you want to do, to getting upset every time you hear a certain tone of voice. Often, these characteristic tendencies that go to make up 'us' are not even consciously *acknowledged*, let alone examined. When we *do* start to notice these patterns, we might also sense that some of them are other than optimal for our well-being – e.g. we seem to constantly argue about household chores with family, we 'sneak out' at night to buy and eat chocolate bars, which we pretend we're buying for friends, etc. Once we have awareness about our patterns, we can start to work on shifting the ones that don't serve us and making more positive, healthy choices.

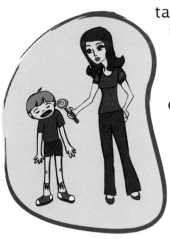

There are many ways in which habitual patterns can be set up. In terms of eating, our parents/guardians may have used food as a 'reward' or to pacify us when upset. We learn to use food, especially things like candies, cookies, cakes and so on, to help us 'feel better' or numb the pain (even if, perversely, these highly processed, addictive foods are the very things that cause us the most damage ultimately).

Other patterns around eating might be set up in a family structure where you *'have'* to finish everything on the plate, regardless of whether or not you are hungry. (Do manipulative statements about how others worldwide are starving sound familiar? Or the request to finish the meal 'to make Mummy happy'?).

Children often learn to eat obediently for acceptance and love. Others may have grown up in a climate of 'lack', afraid that there wasn't enough food to go around. Hence, many of us have deeply entrenched emotional patterns around food, stretching far back into our childhoods, which we still tend to act out now, as adults. We may not even remember specific incidents that helped us create these patterns, yet the power of them is still clearly visible in our current choices, when we choose to look more closely.

When we do focus on the foods we have been choosing to eat, frequently we find that they are processed and de-vitalised. These 'dead' foods are directly intertwined with our 'deadened' emotions. Through our food choices, we have helped numb ourselves to our true potential for vibrant living. The great news is that this can all change. In this book, we explore the deeper aspects of these patterns and aim to turn things around.

I do prefer, though, not to get into much of an analytical 'head-space' in regards to these emotional/spiritual issues. They are delicate in nature, not areas that seem to benefit from intense scrutiny under a harsh spotlight. Trying to intellectualise and fragment matters of the heart and soul doesn't appeal to me; however, I do feel that it's useful to understand *something* of what you're dealing with in the beginning, to help you tune in and allow healing to begin. So, any information shared here that seems a tad 'intellec-tual' is simply to help you get an understanding of the possible dynamics at play in your own life. Then you're free to drop the head-space, get into your heart and allow your delicious recovery to unfold, piece by piece...

Whole Well-Being

This book primarily focuses on the *emotional healing* that a raw food life-style can bring. However, we also touch on many aspects of recovery that might be considered more spiritual/mental/psychological in nature. I see all of these areas as intricately interlinked. It is challenging to separate something as being specific to only one level of our healing, because we are whole beings, simultaneously operating at many levels. For example, your

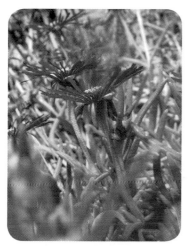

emotional life is not separate from your spiritual or mental life, or your physical body. They all interact and affect each other, just as one simple sentence may affect you in many different ways, on many levels of your being.

I give primary attention here to our emotions, as I see them as the principal guiding system for our lives and something to which most of us can easily relate. Our emotions are like our **navigation system**, letting us know how we feel in any situation: Happy? Sad? Threatened? Excited? Without acknowledging and responding to our emotions, it is less easy to live a stable, happy and 'connected' life.

While most people seem to readily accept that they have emotions and feel-ings – an 'emotional life' – the notion of their own individual 'spirituality' may seem less clear and somehow remote. For me, spirituality is in essence our deeper sense of 'connectedness' to all of life - and it is *this* that primarily underscores the level of joy and peace we experience.

Our emotions in any moment are an expression of how we are feeling, *in connection* to what seems to be happening around us. When we experience a strong, loving, spiritual connection to all of life, we are likely to feel good a great deal of the time, aware of the 'bigger picture' and the fact that ulti-mately, all is well. We have a sense of peace and serenity, regardless of what may appear to be happening in our lives. I'm aware that for some, this might all sound 'far out' and obscure – and may even offend a person who feels that their suffering is 'inevitable'. For this reason, we are going to briefly ex-amine the nature and possibilities of spiritual healing here, before we delve into the main arena of emotional well-being.

Spiritual Healing

If you carry uncomfortable associations with organised religion, it may be that you assume 'spiritual' to be a synonym for 'religious' and defensively back away from this area of transformation. Or perhaps you identify strongly with a certain form of religion and the idea of 'spirituality' may seem vague and even scary to you. The truth is that spiritual recovery is ultimately about *reconnecting to and nurturing our souls* – the deepest, simplest and tru-est parts of *ourselves*. Our spiritual life does not need to be a distant and threatening concept and we certainly do not need to be conventionally 'reli-gious' people to lead spiritual lives. We all have our *own* direct connection to 'Source' from within, even if we can't sense it right now.

When we re-establish the strong soul connection that we knew as children – a connection that was, in most cases, swiftly smothered out by social con-ditioning – we rediscover serenity from within. We can move away from judgements, notions of what seems 'wrong', 'bad' or 'unacceptable' and instead be with what *is*, with loving compassion. We find ourselves content and at peace with the world, regardless of what is going on around us. Any previous misery, anger, self-pity and fear can give way to genuine joy, love, compassion, humility and gratitude.

Can conscious choices made *now* help us move away from subconscious conditioning from the past? Definitely. Again, I feel like I'm living proof.

Some spiritual principles for living that we can begin to examine and integrate include assuming responsibility for our actions, uncondi- tionally accepting ourselves and the world around us, experienc- ing each moment of each day fully and having faith in a 'Greater Power'.

Some of us, of course, stall at the notion of a Greater Power, although this concept is usually quite central in developing spirituality. It means living in the awareness and trust that there is *something* more powerful than we are, beyond these little human structures that we embody. Exactly what you call this thing that represents to you the Greater Power is of little ultimate con- sequence – you might say 'God', 'Buddha', 'Spirit', 'Goddess', 'Great One', 'Universe'. You may even choose to put your faith directly into the power of nature, or a support group you attend, as something more powerful than 'just you'. It really doesn't matter *what* you call this Greater Power; the key is having faith that *something* more powerful than you exists, which can sup- port your journey.

For me, terms like 'God', 'Nature', 'Spirit' and so on are all interchangeable. I feel relaxed with all of them and they seem, to me, to represent the same thing. I believe we are all connected and that the more we get into a direct relationship with nature, the more easy it is to appreciate and feel that uni- ty. I see each one of us as a little spark of light connected within the whole glorious field of being. Our little spark of 'Spirit' is directly connected as a part of the Spirit and flow of the whole Universe – the Greater Power.

Many of us have grown up with negative concepts of a cruel and punishing 'God' who is unforgiving, vengeful and judgemental. As we recover spiritu- ally, we can learn to develop new views of a loving, caring and nurturing Greater Power of our own understanding, to which we are intimately linked. Of course, this doesn't mean that we hand everything over to that Greater Power and sit back on our laurels, expecting everything to automatically be dandy. We have our part to play too, through *action* – by picking up nour- ishing foods to eat, for example, or demonstrating our commitment to our transformation through nourishing daily activities such as reading, writing and sharing with others. Yet I've learned that our Greater Power – if asked – will take care of a great deal. Finding and developing conscious contact with our Greater Power doesn't have to be a scary and distant prospect. Neither do we need anyone else as an intermediary between ourselves and the 'divine'. Direct and meaningful contact is just a short prayer or affirmation away, dissolving our fears with love, hope and courage.

Spiritual recovery is vital for feeling genuinely at peace. If you are holding any defences about this, try to soften and release them. For some of us, entering into a spiritual path may feel frightening and potentially solitary; we might anticipate little support from 'mainstream' society. However, you are always free to stretch out, beyond your own or others' fears and limitations. Rest assured that even if it seems that few people are living a 'spiritual path' in your immediate environment, you are not alone. (If you are on the raw food journey, there are plenty of friends in cyberspace to exchange with, for example – check the resources section for wonderful sites such as www.GiveItToMeRaw.com.)

Raw Food and Spirituality

Eating live, raw, healthy food is considered by many to be an important element in spiritual development. So, if you're already eating mostly raw foods, you're quite probably already on your way to a more in-tune spiritual life. When we stop eating foods such as processed starches, gluten and refined sugar, which block up the body and cloud the brain, we experience a clearing of energy and are more able to connect directly and truthfully to our true essence. Natural and universal laws re-enter our lives with abundance. There is nothing 'mystical' about this - it is just about simplicity.

Many people on dedicated spiritual paths, such as yogis, have simple, high-raw lifestyles. It's even asserted by some that Jesus was a raw foodist. In *The Essene Gospel of Peace*, a reputedly omitted part of the Bible, Jesus says, 'If you eat living food, the same will quicken you, but if you kill your food, the dead food will kill you also.'

The connection between raw food and spirituality is simple: when we live humbly and respectfully from the produce given directly from the Earth, without trying to modify or 'improve' it in some way, we come into alignment with the rest of nature. It is an expression of our commitment to truth and demonstrates our understanding that everything is provided for us, directly from nature.

Through honestly living the path of your highest truth, you will come to see the inter-connectedness of all things, which is an extraordinarily releasing experience. The evidence of your own **metamorphosis** will shine like a beacon for others, with whom you can share your strength and hope as an 'Active Transformer' in your community. Above all, learn to let go and seek to reconnect to that 'small, still voice within' which merges with your Greater Power as a unified guide, helping you surrender into the flow.

Feeling stable in your spiritual life is all about finding balance, as with most aspects of our lives. Engage in regular activities that help you to feel connected and in time you'll come to feel steadier, regardless of any apparent external circumstances. You'll feel more in tune with that which is eternal. This gradual softening into your own spiritual life can be considered easier to handle in many ways than any kind of 'sudden enlightenment' experience, which can be very shocking to the system. Think of this as you might any other areas of change: sudden, huge swings are tough to integrate. Imagine, for example, if your entire physical detox unfolded overnight, or *all* your emotional shifts burst out of you in the space of a few hours. This would be a little intense, yes?

Take a little time every day to nurture the 'spiritual' part of you and you'll come to feel less rushed and stressed, more grounded and more **connected** to who you really are. This book is loaded with great tips to help you with that process – check out the main 'Guidance' section below in particular. Rather than feeling like you're splashing around in an ocean of confusion and anxiety, barely treading water, you'll come to feel like you're *riding* the glorious waves of your own unfolding.

Finding Balance

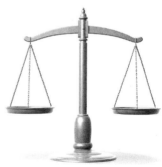

What we are aiming for when examining our emotional and spiritual interactions with food is to find a happy BALANCE, in all areas. Many of us lead fast-paced lives that feel hectic, stressful and almost out of control.
Our relationship with food and the choices we make often form a large part of that feeling of chaos. With the insights and tools offered here for you to use on your own journey, you can find a place of gentle moderation and serenity.

In this book, you will be lovingly guided through a process of transformation. Firstly, you are invited to make an honest appraisal of your current situation, noting anything that seems 'out of balance' with how you'd really love to be living. Then you can choose nourishing *new* habits for yourself, using the many healing tips provided here. As you set about creating a truly balanced, fulfilling lifestyle for yourself, please consider this book your dear friend and ally in this process.

It is possible to release your past destructive patterns with grace and embrace a brighter, lighter life – I did it.

> *"Courage: the power to let go of the familiar."*
> *--Raymond Lindquist*

Focus, Focus, Focus...Where Is Yours?

It is a simple truth that our attention is always focused towards *something*. Our experiences are shaped by *what* it is that we choose to focus our energies on and also how we *feel* in response to those things. Many people end up with rather lop-sided attention patterns, mostly focused on the same things, with their *feelings* towards those things being frequently other than joyful. A typical example might be someone who gives most of their attention to their cigarette breaks from a job they don't enjoy and watches TV programmes with scenes of violence. Similarly, a food addict's attention is usually narrowly focused on food: how to get it, when to eat it, with whom and so on. Both these people have the same opportunities as anyone else in any given moment to focus their attention towards something else. Yet, over and over again, they choose to focus on the same things, even if those things bring little genuine satisfaction and actually damage their well-being. If we learn instead to re-focus our attention so that we're exposed to a broader range of more gentle, nourishing possibilities, we can create more balance and enjoyment for ourselves. We can learn to ease away from and drop the intense, introverted attachment to particular things.

Narrow, fixated 'life patterns' can often emerge from a childhood where positive options either are not present or very limited. It is especially beneficial for children to grow up seeing adults who have a few different healthy interests they enjoy, rather than those who seem to be inflexibly directed towards just one or two aspects of life (e.g. gambling and buying clothes). This doesn't have to mean that we abandon passion and instead live some kind of wishy-washy, 'goody-two-shoes' bland version of life; it just means freedom from a lop-sided and overly intense relationship with certain things.

Your attention is always going towards *something*, in every single moment (even if it's just the 'empty' space of meditation) and there will be a *feeling* associated with that focus.

Do You Choose To Focus On Things That Help You Feel Good?

How would you like to feel? Do you choose a narrow, intense, isolating focus on something like eating junk food, which could ultimately destroy you? Or

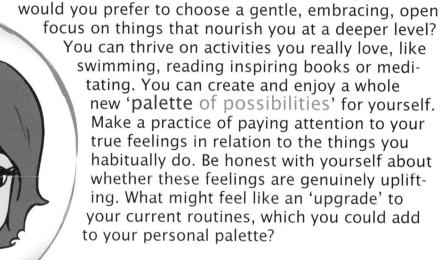

would you prefer to choose a gentle, embracing, open focus on things that nourish you at a deeper level? You can thrive on activities you really love, like swimming, reading inspiring books or meditating. You can create and enjoy a whole new 'palette of possibilities' for yourself. Make a practice of paying attention to your true feelings in relation to the things you habitually do. Be honest with yourself about whether these feelings are genuinely uplifting. What might feel like an 'upgrade' to your current routines, which you could add to your personal palette?

If no positive alternatives immediately spring to mind, your main 'Guidance' section contains plenty of juicy suggestions for you. You can use these to build up an abundant inner fund of what feel like healthier and more fulfilling choices.

How can you easily tell if your relationship to something is a little out of balance? If the thought of it being no longer in your picture sends you into panic, fear, depression or a sense of 'pointlessness', this suggests a strong attachment, which you may benefit from loosening up a little.

It's important here, however, to make a distinction between these slightly sticky, 'toxic' feelings of strong attachment and a passionate involvement with a project that leaves you fulfilled and delighted, even if sometimes a little tired. (Of course, it can sometimes seem hard to distinguish one from the other.)

Say, for example, a friend is creating an event into which he or she focuses a great deal of their time and energy. From the outside looking in, an observer may think that this friend is 'obsessed' with the event, or is a 'workaholic' and that the situation is unhealthy. However, that person might actually be having a mostly fabulous time preparing the event, feeling totally inspired, excited and thrilled to be working on their project. In this case, the *joy* they are experiencing is likely serving the greater good immensely, as they are following their bliss.

The important thing, of course, is not how others interpret you, rather *your* personal understanding of the messages from your own emotions. As I've said, I see our emotions as our guidance system in life - they are *extremely* useful to observe. If we are observant of our feelings and follow our intuition, it is much easier to lead a happy, grounded life, feeling connected to Spirit. Paying attention to our feelings is key, in order to know if something truly brings us pleasure. For example, someone who compulsively eats ice cream may think that they enjoy it, yet if they really give close attention to their feelings before, during and after eating, they might discover a different story. They might see that, in fact, before eating they felt anxious, during they felt frantic and afterwards they felt guilty. Where is the joy?

I believe it is up to each of us to check in with *ourselves* about how we really feel in regards to the things we give attention towards and to seek more balance if that seems beneficial. No-one knows better than you how you genuinely feel about something. This kind of self-reflection and honesty can, however, feel confronting. Fortunately, there are many exercises and suggestions in these pages that can help you.

So...What Does Your Emotional Connection with Food Look Like...?
(...or you think you haven't got one?)

It seems that in our Western societies especially, most of us have quite complex relationships with food. We're going to examine the nature of these emotional attachments here.

The Emotional Connection

The connection between food and mood for humans is generally immense. We eat to celebrate; we eat if we feel sad; we eat to 'reward' ourselves; we eat because someone gives us something and we feel 'obliged'. Ironically, we rarely seem to eat simply to fuel the physical body. Yet we tend to so rarely discuss our strong emotional connections to food. Some people may never even have given it a thought.

Most of us have heard that 'You are what you eat'. In addition to this, I believe that our attitudes, feelings and beliefs about what we're eating are at *least* as important as what we're actually putting in our mouths. We are also *how* and *why* we eat. If we consume food, for example, while feeling something like shame, anger or guilt, this has a BIG impact on the way that food is digested and assimilated into the body. We can learn and heal so much from understanding our emotional connection with food.

Seven Ways of Eating: Keys to Your Understanding

It's fair to say that I've had good reason to reflect on relationships towards food. My curiosity and learning have brought me to see seven main ways in which we seem to relate to and use food. These are marked in green in the diagram below.

This conceptualisation grew from my personal interest. I could see how on the *surface* two people might eat exactly the same meal, yet their *experiences* of eating that food could be completely different. One might thoroughly enjoy it, whereas the other one eats it with guilt and afterwards feels remorse. I wanted to explore what might underscore these different experiences. I came to see that it seemed to be related to two key factors, both their *emotional connection* to food and their amount of focused *consciousness/self-reflection* in regards to eating. The chart below suggests some versions of the interplay of these two factors.

It's my feeling that most of us carry an emotional connection with food to some extent, some more than others. When you take a look at the categories below, you may find that one way of eating describes you; or you might shift from one 'zone' to another, or even feel that you shuttle relentlessly between a few. See where you think you might fit in:

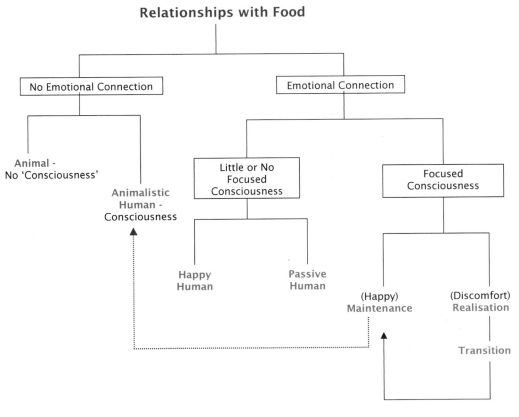

Recognise yourself in any, or a few of these?

'Animal'
- I eat food for physical fuel and that's it. I have no emotional connection to it.
- I have a simple, constant connection to the Universe.
- I don't engage in 'self-reflection'.

'Animalistic Human'
- I eat food for physical fuel. I have no emotional connection to it.
- I have a simple, constant connection to the Universe.
- I engage in self-reflection.

'Happy Human'
- I have an emotional connection to food, though I'm not consciously aware of it. I feel good about my eating.
- I don't engage in self-reflection about my relationship with food.
- I might experience feeling a 'spiritual connection' or might not.

'Passive Human'
- I have an emotional connection to food, though I am not consciously aware of it. I feel unhappy or indifferent about my eating.
- I engage in little to no self-reflection about my relationship with food.
- I might experience feeling a spiritual connection or might not.

'Realisation'
- I recognise my emotional connection to food. I feel discomfort about how things have been going. I'm ready and willing to make some shifts.
- I start to reflect on myself and my relationship with food.
- I am often looking for spiritual connection, consciously or not.

'Transition'
- I'm moving towards a happy emotional connection with food.
- I engage in self-reflection.
- I feel I am reconnecting spiritually.

'Maintenance'
- I feel consistently happy with my emotional life and eating.
- I engage in self-reflection.
- I often feel spiritually connected and content.

These categories are of course a little crude. As I have said, you may not necessarily feel that you fit into only one of these categories and you may also move between them over time. Someone may even fluctuate repeatedly between two or more categories.

This conceptualisation of the different ways in which we can relate to food may help us to generally clarify our current relationship with eating, plus consider shifts we may or may not want to experience. So, let's take a closer look at these different categories.

It seems to me that almost all animals, other than humans, come under the 'Animal' category (or at least the wild animals). They seem to eat purely for physical nourishment. However, I make no claim to know how all those animals feel and perhaps they do experience something of the other stages outlined here.

People within the 'Animalistic Human' category seem to be rather few in numbers to me, at least in the societies I'm used to living in. One well-known example is Anastasia, currently living in the Siberian forests of Russia. Anastasia lives 'wild' in the forest, deeply connected to all around her. She never

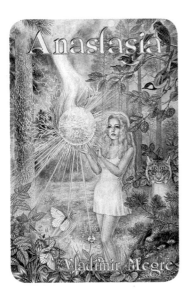

stops to prepare and eat a 'meal'; she simply picks at berries here or nuts there, within the natural course of her days. She is *truly* raw. She seems to have no discernible emotional relationship with food, other than a simple love and appreciation for that which nourishes her. As she puts it, she 'eats just as she breathes'. You can read about Anastasia's life in the profoundly inspiring and educational 'Ringing Cedars' series of books by Vladimir Megré. I imagine that Anastasia's relationship to food and the Earth is similar to many tribal people, worldwide. Traditionally, for example, Australian Aborigines lived nomadically, in close connection to the Earth, taking food with simple reverence, as needed. There was no cultivation of crops, rather, simple appreciation for what is given from the land. In most Western cultures, we have become starkly divorced from this experience of immediate connection.

I sense that most other humans can find themselves described in one or more of the remaining five categories – Happy Humans, Passive Humans, Realisation, Transition and Maintenance. So, what characterises these different relationships with food?

'Happy Humans', often smiling and seemingly content, may eat what on the surface seems like a pretty toxic load for their entire lives and never question their patterns. They *enjoy* the things they eat. This is very important, in the grander scheme. It really seems like the most vital thing, in fact – enjoying our experiences here. These people may be a little overweight; they may *seem* unhealthy and even 'disconnected' spiritually to those observing them and *yet*...they are happy. We've all heard of people who eat what appears to be a other-than-optimal intake, yet live to be 100 or thereabouts; they might be considered Happy Humans. A common trait among those who eat 'other than optimally', yet are long-lived is **moderation**. They commonly eat small amounts, rather than overeating.

Systematic under-eating is one of the major keys for longevity. As raw food author David Wolfe succinctly puts it, 'We have yet to discover an obese centenarian'.

Now, what about the 'Passive Human'? The Passive Human kind of relationship with food seems typically expressed in someone who generally feels down or indifferent about most things in life and is perhaps a little apathetic. They don't feel great about their relationship with food yet engage in little to no self-reflection about it. These people may seem truly stuck in heavy emotions, or, at the very least, experience a sense of 'flatness' and inertia. They may even isolate themselves as recluses, experience ongoing depression and a sense of hopelessness. Their relationship with food is of course just one feature of this state. They are not happy about their relationship with food, yet not uncomfortable enough to begin really examining this and making shifts.

The defining contrast between people in the Happy/Passive Human categories and those in Realisation/Transition/Maintenance is the *degree of focused consciousness* and true self-reflection about our patterns.

The 'Realisation' stage is a key phase, the point at which consciousness really comes in, usually with some sense of discomfort; a feeling that the way we've been living has not been entirely optimal. This is a time of great shifts and awareness. Depending on your background and support, this might expand into a time of major delight, filled with optimism and anticipation, as you start to explore new ideas and ways of living. You may also find that you feel extremely uncomfortable or anxious occasionally. This is prime time to acknowledge whatever it is that you are becoming aware of and feeling. Myriad possibilities are opening to you...

> *"And the day came*
> *when the risk to remain tight in a bud*
> *was more painful than the risk it took to blossom."*
> *--Anaïs Nin*

The 'Transitional' stage is all about *action*. After coming to a place of being willing to *do* something about our relationship with food, we choose our course of action and we *do* it. The length of time we experience this stage largely depends on how quickly our feelings shift into being more-or-less **consistently positive** around our food choices. For example, one person may begin their Transition feeling miserable, start to make positive changes with their food choices, work through their major emotional stumbling blocks and feel genuinely great day by day within a month.

Someone else might go into their Transition and stay cruising about in that category for years. They might find it awkward to consistently move onwards into a happier, more balanced relationship with food. They might stay stuck in their heads about certain emotional issues; they might have problems with completely surrendering certain foods that no longer serve them and may feel uncomfortable about all this.

Others might feel like they wobble backwards and forwards a great deal between being a Passive Human and feeling like they're in Realisation (or even perhaps taking a little action and dipping their toes into Transition). They might move to and fro between apathy and then awareness of what they're doing, yet never quite gain the momentum to take *solid* action. Instead, they may block things out with denial and backslide into that 'Passive' mode again. When they start to feel they're really moving *forwards* with action, choosing foods they feel great about, thinking positively about their choices, enjoying their lives, working through emotional detox and so on, this may be the time they start to recognise themselves more as being truly in Transition. The final category, 'Maintenance', describes people who have come to a place where they feel consistently great about their relationship with eating. They have worked through the more lumpy areas of Transition and have found a stable place of balance in life, with self-reflection and consciousness. Those in 'Maintenance' may not feel great about their food choices in *every* single moment – there may be 'blips' here and there.

However, remember that it's what we do and how we feel *most* of the time rather than the 'blips' that matters here. Someone who is in a Maintenance relationship with food will feel good about his or her food choices *most* of the time.

You might notice on the chart that I have linked the Maintenance category to the Animalistic Human category with a *dotted line.* This is to indicate that those who reach that happy state of Maintenance (perhaps especially if raw foodists) might project their vision beyond Maintenance and aspire to live like an Animalistic Human, such as Anastasia (described above). I know for myself, this is certainly true – Anastasia's apparent absence of an emotional connection with food fascinates and inspires me.

While I believe that, in *theory*, it is entirely possible for someone in Maintenance to become in essence Animalistic Human in their eating style, harmonising this with, for example, a citified life, is a definite challenge. It seems this kind of transformation would more or less necessitate removing oneself from modern cultures, where so much of our identity and society is based around food.

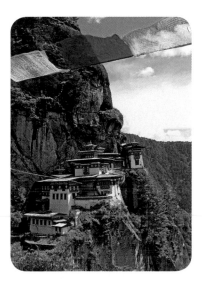

Indeed, you might be wondering how and if people in simpler or 'tribal' communities fit into the 'seven ways of eating' scheme in the chart above.

Let's take, for example, the people of Bhutan, a tiny kingdom in the Himalaya Mountains. Most people there, as in many regions of the world, lead comparatively simple lives, close to nature. They often eat things that are cooked, yet almost everything they eat is a whole food, straight from nature. Bhutan is known as one of the most isolated countries in the world yet also has one of the happiest populations on the planet. The King of Bhutan himself declared that '**Gross National Happiness** is more important than Gross National Product.' The Bhutanese, as a nation, seem like a definite example to me of 'Happy Humans': they eat simple food, live close to the Earth and enjoy a clean, beautiful environment. They are by no means a nation of raw foodists, yet on average they seem to have relatively long, healthy and certainly happy lives. It is also reported that some people (especially monks and yogis) out in the Himalayas live for 120+ years. Perhaps some of these super-centenarians are raw, although most likely not. What they almost certainly share is a positive outlook, 'pristine' air quality, a simple connection to life and a moderate, balanced intake.

If this overview feels helpful to you, you can identify which, if any, of these 'food relationship' categories you feel might apply to you. However, there are two pertinent points to clarify here. Firstly, the purpose of these categories is not to rigidly put yourself into a box, or to chastise yourself if you can't quite fit into any of them. The idea is simply to open our awareness, for the purpose of positive change.

Secondly, these categories are not a yardstick for self-judgement. Some people may stump their own healing by judging themselves by standards/ideas they have seen elsewhere and believe to be correct/acceptable, rather than checking in with *themselves* concerning how they feel about their transformation. For example, someone may read here about life as a balanced raw foodie in 'Maintenance' and keep saying to themselves for years 'no, that's not me, that description doesn't quite fit' and berating themselves for it, whereas in fact, they've come a *huge* way in their transformation and are doing great.

You know your self, your mind and your body best – no-one else. If you feel you are progressing well on your healing path, then that is your truth and it's completely valid, even if it doesn't seem to fit someone else's model. Be sure to acknowledge and validate your own shifts.

The *raw foods* path is, of course, just one option for transforming our relationship with food.

Thousands of people may reach the Realisation stage and choose to enter their Transition with approaches other than going raw. For example, if previously they were eating a Standard American Diet (SAD), they may simply continue to eat the same things, just reducing the quantities, or perhaps they will choose to go vegetarian, or start eating a Macrobiotic diet and so on. We might also find people choosing to eat mainly raw foods within *any* of these seven categories.

This book is aimed primarily towards people who are choosing raw foods with conscious intent and are most likely in the Realisation/Transition stages. My aim is to guide you comfortably towards a state of happy Maintenance. While there are countless ways to re-model our relationships with food, raw food (for me), represents the most simple, yet revolutionary and truly connected route available. I also feel it is the most optimal way to eat for physical health in the human body. That is why I love it so much and why I support others in choosing this path.

Where Consciousness Comes In

Let's consider that, at first glance, people in the Happy Human and Maintenance categories could potentially be observed eating exactly the same thing – let's say a cheese sandwich. Both feel happy about it and get on with their day. Is there a difference? Why might we consider these two people as being in different 'categories'?

The principal difference here is the focused *consciousness* behind the action. The person who is in Maintenance has worked through a (frequently long and rocky) emotional healing process, from Realisation, through Transition, to a point where they feel genuinely happy and at peace with their choices. They've put a lot of attention on healing their relationship with food, to get to this balanced place of Maintenance; they display focus, consciousness and self-reflection in their eating patterns.

The Happy Human, on the other hand, has never *stopped* feeling good about their food choices. In fact they may never really *consider* their emotional connection to food and might even be described as 'oblivious' to these concerns. They do not *consciously* focus on these matters, as it's simply 'no big deal' to them. They are perfectly happy as they are.

So, when these two people both eat a cheese sandwich, on the *surface* they may seem to an observer to have the same kind of relationship with food – i.e., they eat something and seem to feel content about it. Yet the *back-*

ground of how they each came to that point of happiness might be very different, as well as the feelings/perceptions/thoughts/experiences that each actually has before, during or after eating.

The Happy Human might make and eat the cheese sandwich for lunch, just as they have every day for the last fifteen years, feel their usual sense of contentment and get on with their day. The person in Maintenance might be working with a daily Food Plan (see pgs. 124 - 128) that they would check regarding what they intended to eat for lunch, make the sandwich, feel grateful that they're eating this and not a greasy hamburger instead, bless their food, enjoy the meal and then make a conscious effort after eating to step away from the kitchen and get on with other things, rather than potentially eating more. There is more awareness directed to their internal processes. It is also *quite* likely that someone who has gone through the whole recovery process, to arrive in the Maintenance category will be eating less food and *different* foods than the Happy Human. Naturally, some people in Maintenance are even 100% raw.

Compared to the Happy Human, who never *stopped* feeling good about his or her relationship with food, the person who is in Maintenance may sometimes find it more of an issue to maintain **positive feelings** about food. As we've learned, many in Maintenance have been through a long healing

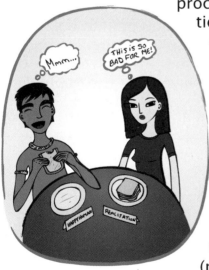

process to reach that point - they have more emotional 'scar tissue' than a Happy Human, which can be stirred up at times. It is vital, though, for people in Maintenance to let go of any old attachments and focus on the *present* moment, to really maintain and enjoy peace of mind. If you feel you are in Maintenance and yet find yourself unexpectedly getting tied up thinking things like 'is it really okay if I eat this?', 'what will other people think if they see me eating this?' or 'am I going to mess everything up if I eat this extra slice of apple?', it might be a wise time to relax and review some of the suggestions for those in Maintenance later in this book (pgs. 217-226).

We can also play around with comparing the above cheese-sandwich-eating experience of a Happy Human or someone in Maintenance to a person in any of the Passive Human, Realisation or Transition stages. Eating a cheese sandwich could feel like a catastrophe to someone in one of those latter stages, depending on their situation on that particular day. It is therefore not just the food itself that influences our health and well-being, but also our *feelings* about what we are eating. Do you see how two people could be eating exactly the same thing and have a completely different experience with it? Everybody's actions are guided by some set of beliefs – what are yours?

If you find it tricky to understand the concept that consciousness could make such a big difference for someone's health and connection with food, please consider the following more extreme example.

Think about the difference between someone being held in a concentration camp, who has very little or nothing to eat and is withering away, compared to a breatharian, who is living on basically air and water and is in prime health. At first glance, both people are consuming almost exactly the same things, yet where one is thriving, the other is barely surviving. What is the difference here? Well, while there may of course be many, many other underlying factors to consider, one key difference seems, to me, to be the consciousness around their 'food' consumption.

Whereas the breatharian has made the conscious choice to live in this way and is enjoying the experience, the person in the concentration camp most likely feels terrible. Here, consciousness can ultimately mean the huge difference between living and dying. It is also a matter of pace of adaptation: the breatharian has chosen to take this path, which involves a conscious preparation process that was likely engaged at his or her own pace over a long period of time. The person in the concentration camp, on the other hand, has likely seen a dramatic, unanticipated shift in their life, rather than a slow adaptation. This could be compared to the difference between training yourself to hold your breath underwater for long periods of time or being suddenly forced to do so because someone is holding your head underwater. Each person has an entirely different emotional/conscious disposition in the 'same' circumstance.

Ideally this section has given you a clearer picture of how our emotions and consciousness might inter-relate and help characterise our eating patterns. Perhaps you've even identified yourself somewhere in the diagram above. With that in mind, we're now going to shine the spotlight back down the track a little, to see where we're coming from in terms of emotional 'health', especially in relation to our eating habits...

How HAVE You Been Dealing With Your Emotions?

Putting a Lid On It?

Ask most people how they feel and what do they say? 'Fine', 'Great', 'Good, thanks'. If you look a little below the surface, however, the truth is frequently quite different from what these automatic 'polite' responses suggest. This is a simple example of how people seem to lose connection to their genuine feelings. It's as if there's an assumption that it's only acceptable to present the world with a positive response, no matter how insincere it may be compared to your actual emotional state. In fact, many of us are so embroidered in our own complicated emotional webs that we no longer even *know* how we truly feel. All we do know is that we want to present a 'good image' to the world. We want (consciously or unconsciously) to be accepted.

Growing up in a family where it seems 'unacceptable' to be sad or angry, or to express real feelings, children may learn to keep their truth quiet and instead present a 'happy' face to the world, a habit they carry into adulthood. The real emotions get internalised instead, to deal with at some later point. We co-create a society of individuals who are pretty 'toxic' emotionally, sometimes filled to bursting point with troubles and issues that are blithely glossed over with a friendly 'fine, thanks'. Here, the 'outer' grossly misrepresents the 'inner'.

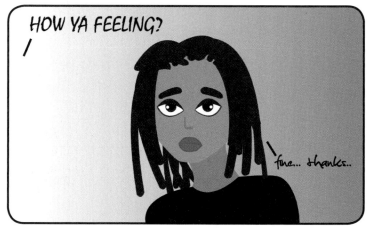

These suppressed emotions do not simply go away when they are not expressed or released. They stay in the emotional energy body of the person and may seek expression in any number of ways. Feelings of hurt, anger, loneliness, wrath and so on that may underlie the 'fine, thanks' response commonly get released as sarcasm, gossiping or complaining. Also, people frequently assume 'roles' (e.g. people-pleaser or group clown) to deal with their emotional disconnection. They may use substances like drugs, alcohol or *foods* as a form of escape, or reach 'breaking point' and go into raging emotional outbursts. It seems like a far healthier approach to learn to embrace your emotions and simply express them *as they arise*, rather than dealing with unhealthy outlets for your *suppressed* feelings further down the line. (We examine more deeply how emotional issues can manifest in our lives, *beyond* our eating patterns, in the 'Introduction to Emotional Detox' and 'Releasing' sections, which run back-to-back from pages 134-161.)

Digestion As Diversion

The fact is that it takes a lot of energy to process our emotions; it also takes a lot of energy to digest foods (especially manufactured, unnatural 'foods'). Hence, a common way that people avoid going into their emotional truth is by 'eating over' any strong feelings that surface, to squash the feeling back down. This way, the primary flow of their energy is diverted into digesting the contents of their stomach rather than processing their emotions. When we 'eat over' our feelings like this, we can numb out once again, stuffing the feelings down, to be dealt with at some other time.

This can be likened to **suppressing** *physical* symptoms that are seeking release, with allopathic medicines (e.g. using antibiotics to 'cure' a rash). It may seem as though you've found a quick solution, yet in the long term, this unreleased toxicity will surely and simply resurface to be released in another form, while, in the meantime, you have just added more to your body's toxic load with the intake of antibiotics.

The same thing happens with any emotions we 'stuff down'. We might 'self-medicate' ourselves with food (diverting our energy into digestion) and feel, either consciously or unconsciously, that we have managed today's little emotional hump. Yet those feelings don't just disappear; they too get backed up in our systems, often 'poisoning' us from within. Many of us harbour a quagmire of unresolved emotions; we might feel misunderstood, unappreciated, unable to relate to others and so on. These unexpressed emotions come up for release too and may seek expression in sudden emotional outbursts, nervous breakdowns, hysterical laughing fits and so on. In the meantime, we've once again added to the toxic load of our bodies by using unnatural foods and excess food as our 'suppressant'.

Different people handle emotional intensity in different ways. Consider, as an example, someone who has an interview coming up that is very important to them. That person might feel so anxious about the interview that they 'can't eat'; their energy is so wrapped up in the tension of anticipation that their appetite shuts down. They are busy processing *emotions* and have no interest in digesting food. In contrast, another person in the same situation might react in an apparently opposite way. As feelings of stress and nervousness arise about the interview, they seem to automatically reach for the cookie jar or ice cream carton, to stuff those feelings down, divert their energy into digestion instead and numb out.

 Sometimes, if we do eat at the same time that we're trying to process intense emotions, we might end up with a feeling of nausea, indigestion or similar discomfort. It is simply all too much for the body to handle at once. In these instances, it is often wise to calm yourself down into a place of balance and stillness, so that your body can work more easily on the digestion first. You might do some very gentle yoga, sit in meditation, breathe deeply, go for a relaxing walk in nature or watch an uplifting film; choose something to help *shift* the focus from your emotions for a while, so that your body can first complete the digestion process more easily. You can always return your focus to your emotional unfoldment later on; you may even be relieved to find that the intensity has also lessened, while you've had your attention elsewhere.

As we travel the path of our transformation, we may reach a point where we are eating regularly, calmly, consistently and with no big 'wobbles' in any direction. We feel balanced. Then, all of a sudden, BAM, some kind of stress appears in our life and we might find ourselves diving straight back into the cookie jar. It is a common pattern. Some people feel so stressed, edgy and un-peaceful *most* of the time that their lives literally lurch from one kind of binge to another. This seems to be especially typical among city-dwellers with fast-paced, hectic lives; there is little sense of inner calm or connectedness.

When we go raw, this whole dynamic between processing emotions and digesting food can flip dramatically.

At the start, most people tend to eat quite heavy, dense, gourmet raw foods and large quantities. Yet even so, this is generally a vast improvement on our previous intake. In this stage you might feel very excited, euphoric even, exploring your new path; it is like a 'honeymoon' period, where we feel relief and hope, as we release our relationship with toxic foods. However, as time passes, we usually start to eat lighter raw foods and smaller quantities, which means less work for the digestive system. In terms of our emotions, this means there is progressively more space and energy available for our feelings to be released. For most, this is truly a new way of interacting with 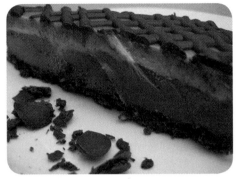 the world and can feel quite intense. We go deeper and deeper into detox, on every level. Many people simply do not want to delve into this level of emotional detox and will either eat many heavy/dense raw foods to try to compensate, or yo-yo back and forth between cooked and raw. Some may simply turn away from raw foods altogether.

After the initial glow of the honeymoon period fades, we typically find that our *underlying* issues are still there, below the surface, looking to be released. If we are not ready and willing to process our emotions as they come up, this new lifestyle can begin to feel challenging or uncomfortable. Compared to how things were when we ate 'comfort' foods, it might now feel like we're living with a deficit. At least back then, things felt comfortable and familiar, even if we weren't that happy. Now we're eating new healthier foods and we're *still* not happy – in fact it feels like there are even more issues to deal with and nowhere familiar to hide, as the safety net of 'comfort foods' has gone. It is at times like these that your mind may readily chime in with thoughts like 'forget this eating healthy stuff; let's go back to candy, that was more fun!'. Hence, the wobble back to familiarity often follows, even if *logically* you know that those old familiar foods are not better for you. In the face of strong emotional detox, without solid support and focus, it is remarkably common for people to relapse into their old habits.

To sidestep these potential pitfalls, I *strongly* recommend inquiring into your *emotional* unfoldment on this journey just as lovingly as you channel energy into your new food choices. That's what this book is here to help you do, so I'm glad to see that you're still reading!

Consciousness Enters

Some people live their whole lives in a bubble of suppressed and unexpressed emotions and never really do anything about it. They would tend to fall into our 'Happy' and 'Passive' Human categories. Obviously, the Happy ones feel mostly fine about their experiences, whereas the Passive ones may range from apathetic to chronically depressed. The key difference between these people and those in our other categories, as we have explored, is focused *consciousness*.

It is the point at which consciousness really enters our lives – the Realisation stage – that clearly-seen issues can arise. We start to examine the way we connect emotionally to ourselves, others, food and so on and...we feel discomfort in some way. People often arrive at the Realisation stage at a point in their lives when they feel as if they've 'hit rock bottom'. Perhaps they've reached a weight they never thought they'd see on their scales, or they just can't face going on another diet. In my case, a diabetes scare was the turning point for me that pushed me into Realisation. For many of us, it takes facing that kind of extreme discomfort to blow open our awareness and launch us into what is sometimes a 'do-or-die' Realisation.

With the conscious awareness Realisation brings, we may finally see how we've been using *food* as an escape hatch, to stuff down our emotions and diffuse our stress. These patterns that until now seemed to be serving us suddenly feel like a toxic blanket covering over the truth that lies within. We don't want to keep covering up. We want out. We don't want to keep eating these toxic foods that numb us. We want to feel a genuine connection to ourselves and others. Sometimes that feels inspiring and freeing. Yet it can still feel very daunting too, to step into unknown territory...

My Own Experience

I underwent a dramatic transformation emotionally as I began to heal. Prior to adopting this lifestyle, I was really quite a caustic, controlling and angry person. I read through old diaries of mine from those days with absolute shock. I was so bitter, resentful and sarcastic. My focus was nearly always on 'negative' aspects of life. Everything was a 'problem' in some way and people everywhere left me irritated. I swore a lot. I exaggerated. I lied. I would gossip behind peoples' backs. I felt filled with destruction and violence (surely not unrelated to the toxic, processed factory meat products and other 'foods' made without love that I consumed in vast quantities daily).

I mostly hid my emotional toxicity from public view. On the surface, I tried to maintain some kind of mask of being 'the good girl', the straight-A student, the people-pleaser, while inside I was raging. I absolutely never cried in public and a few people later told me that they found me quite cold, unapproachable and even 'scary' during this time of my life...wow... At the time, though, I had no idea that the way I was living was so fear-based. I can see with hindsight and compassion that I was an extremely lonely, depressed, fearful, obese teenager. At the time, I thought I was hilarious and completely justified in my anger. Perversely, I also believe that if you'd asked me then if I was happy in life, I would almost certainly have said 'yes' and have more or less believed that. I simply didn't know at that time that there was any other way. Consciousness about my emotional patterns had not yet entered the picture for me.

> "Nothing will benefit human health and increase chances of survival for life on Earth as much as the evolution to a vegetarian diet."
> --Albert Einstein

I am very happy to say that my emotional life now is markedly different. These days I am genuinely happy in life. I focus on positivity and enjoyment as much as possible. I feel stable, serene and content most of the time. I meditate, pray and send loving, healing thoughts out daily to those I sense will benefit from them. In more recent years, one of the phrases that has resonated the most for me is that 'vulnerability is my greatest defence'. The first time I heard this, I felt a huge wave of relief wash over me. It felt so very true. I saw that there was no 'need' for me to wear any kind of mask towards the world, hide my tears or shroud my fears. It is not necessary to pretend to be anything other than that which I am; I can share my true feelings, freely and happily. This feels immensely liberating.

I will not say that I live in an emotional nirvana now, where all is blissfully happy in every single moment. I certainly have challenging times and dark moments too. Yet I know that I have a choice in every moment as to how I feel. Most of the time, I choose to feel good. I embrace a sense of wonder. It is all a process, as the emotional journey unfolds for me with grace. Just like the physical detox can be thought of as 'never-ending', as we clean out more and more layers of generations-old waste, the same is true at the emotional level. It seems there is always more to unfold, like peeling away the layers

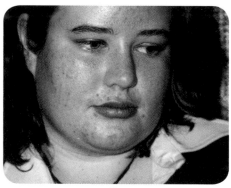

Before

of an onion. So, while I certainly wouldn't say that my emotional journey has reached any kind of 'completion' (or likely ever will), I am very happy with the current state of my emotional well-being, especially when compared to how I used to feel.

How did I get from that toxic, bitter, warped state, to my current happy and grateful state of being? Well, it was a big journey for me and I used many tools along the way, including most of those listed in this book's 'Guidance' section. For me, the beginning stages of my transformation felt particularly disruptive, like my life was turning inside out. I felt anxious, exposed, bitter and fearful. I just wanted to get out, to the other side - I didn't want to deal with the release of old stuff or learning new ways of handling my emotions. I just wanted it all to feel OK. It was an enormous step for me to learn to share my truth with others about what was happening for me. Prior to this, I had rarely spoken my truth to anyone - I was very secretive. I took it day by day though, breathed deeply and found that slowly I moved through the pain and towards the light, as I opened up more and more. These days I am delighted that I experience so much more integrity, openness and FUN in my life. My inner and outer are in alignment. I feel a genuine connection to my feelings, which are like my guidance system. Now, if someone asks me how I feel, they can expect an honest answer...

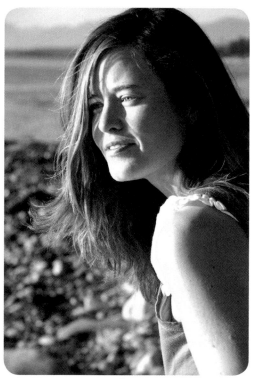

After

Food As a Crutch

One of the main coping mechanisms we use to mask and suppress our emotions is food. When we take the chance to look a little closer, the relationship we have had with *whatever* we've chosen to numb ourselves with can feel quite toxic (e.g. alcohol, TV, shopping) – and food is no exception.

We may have come to depend on food as our crutch for dealing with different situations. Our eating may be compulsive; a great deal of our time and energy may be focused on food and we may end up heavily overweight and

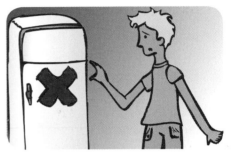

feeling out of control. As with any addiction, we're using the food to try to help us change our *mood*. This can be considered at root a spiritual malady. We're attempting to fill a void inside ourselves. Yet that void cannot be filled by something physical. That void stems from a loss of connection with our true self. It is a void that yearns to be filled with an authentic, loving emotional and spiritual connection – not more

corn chips. Ironically, we use the food as our crutch to try to help us fill the aching hole inside and feel better, yet in truth, we are pulling our health and well-being further into decline, as our cells expand with toxic waste and our hearts and souls remain yearning for sincere expression. We are reaching out and grabbing something to heal us that simply doesn't suit the job.

The answer is not in the fridge ;)

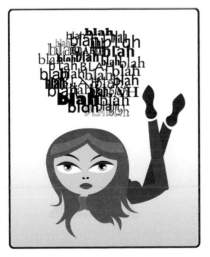

At heart, we are simple beings. We all long to be loved, to feel happy and enjoy our experiences. However, on top of that simple, loving, child-like core, many people in our societies tend to end up with a tangled pile of complicated stories, beliefs, patterns, habits, fears and memories. The simple, loving core inside – the little flickering light that longs to be seen and to share – gets smothered and blocked out. Instead of coming from a space of love, we start to operate from a place of fear. We might feel lost, isolated, abandoned, victimised. Or we might feel resentful, bitter, competitive and angry. We might take on *roles* to try to gain the feeling of love and connection we so yearn for: perhaps we become an 'overachiever', a 'people-pleaser' or a 'hero'. Many of us, though, turn to food as our ally. Food feels safe. It is legal, it doesn't argue back or judge us. It helps us feel physically full, it can help sedate us with compounds like the opioids in wheat products, plus it is acceptable and often even *encouraged* to consume lots of food socially.

It is the point at which a person starts to feel *uneasy* about their relationship with food that things can really get stirred up. If someone shifts into the Realisation category, they may go from feeling comfort, thrill or joy around eating, to the realisation that the way they're eating is other than optimal for vibrant health. The feeling changes. The 'buzz' they got from eating is no longer anywhere near the same. It may be replaced with grief, remorse, disgust, fear and anxiety. They may feel stuck. Upon reflection, the reliance on food as a crutch suddenly seems toxic and the relationship with this 'ally' becomes an undesirable drain. It can be physically destructive, socially isolating and leave us feeling emotionally and spiritually disconnected. Besides the physical addiction to certain foods, a huge emotional bond has also been created. If that goes, what is the food addict going to be left with? This is a fear that keeps most overeaters hooked to their 'drug' of choice, long after the food has ceased to feel exciting or comforting. Yet we *can* transform our patterns into something new and healthier if we choose to – it is just a matter of conscious choice.

To read this far suggests to me that you are likely in either the Realisation stage or Transitional – great places to be. It's equally great to simply be curious and enquiring into creating shifts, at whichever stage of the game you feel you are.

Realisation
The Realisation stage can be one of great revelation. This is the point at which we become conscious of and ACKNOWLEDGE (even if just to ourselves) our emotional connection with food. Self-reflection leads us to become willing to make shifts. Feelings may range wildly at this point, from excitement and delight to isolation, confusion and fear.

Transition
The Transitional stage of our transformation is all about ACTION. Intellectual education on a subject is useful to an extent, yet it's feel-

ing *inspired*, making a real *commitment* and taking *action* that brings actual results. During Transition, we actively seek healthy balance in our choices, as well as support for this new lifestyle, as we reach out to others on a similar path.

OK, So I Eat – Does That Mean I'm Addicted?

Quite likely, if you OVER-eat – or if you are 'fixed' on certain foods and feel that you can't tug yourself away. So, what is behind the compulsion to 'act out' with food? There are two main aspects to addiction – physiological and/ or psychological. An addiction might be based in one or the other of these, or a bit of both...

Physiological Addiction: shows up in the experience of physical withdrawal symptoms such as headaches, shakiness, fatigue, etc., when you stop using the addictive substance – e.g. alcohol, cigarettes, drugs.

Psychological Addiction: a dependency of the mind – shows up in psychological withdrawal symptoms like cravings, irritability and depression, when you stop the activity. Examples might be shopping, exercise, computers, pornography, religion.

Gambling, for example, can be considered a 'psychological addiction' – there is nothing the person is physically taking into their body. These kinds of addictions can also be thought of as psycho-social behavioural disorders.

Compulsive (over)eating of highly processed foods, however, has both psychological *and* physiological elements. 'Foods' like processed starches, refined sugars and coffee are highly addictive at the physical level. On top of this, people get hooked on using those foods for comfort and escape and so they form behavioural (psychological) patterns of use, which are then tricky to turn around.

In the beginning, most addictions bring the user some sense of pleasure: food, alcohol, cigarettes. Over time, however, the person's body becomes so full of toxins that at any point in which they are *not* ingesting their 'drug of choice', they are going into detox/withdrawal from it, which feels painful. The compulsion to keep using their chosen substance hence becomes less about the immediate pleasure it brings and more about plain relief from the pain of detox/withdrawal. In terms of food addiction, people don't want to feel the pain of detox (consciously or unconsciously), so they keep eating the addictive foods. They are physically dependent on them and their bodies rapidly start to break down into disease as a result of ingesting so many toxins.

> *"The more frequent the indulgence, the stronger the craving*
> *but less the appreciation."*
> *--Dr. Ann Wigmore*

The Physiological Addiction

The things I was eating as 'food' in my obese days were so processed that, with hindsight, it's not surprising that I was addicted to such 'Franken-food' concoctions. I was caught in a sticky web of wheat, sugars, refined salt and starches. How did I get into that web? Healthy children do not naturally start to reach out for bread, cakes or hamburgers; they are mainly interested in fruits. Eating **Franken-foods** like these is learned behaviour. Most of us are actually exposed to addictive foods like refined sugars from *pre-birth*, while we're still in the womb. Then, after passing our first few months post-birth being raised usually on breast milk (which is frequently packed with toxins from the mother) or 'formula' milk powder, we are trained to start eating processed baby food. For most of us, it's a spiral into more and more toxicity from there. By the time we reach adulthood, we're thoroughly 'hooked on cooked' toxins and immersed in our emotional dependency on them; it's easy to see why it might feel challenging to let go and choose something different to eat.

So, what's in these toxic foods that we get addicted to? What stimulates the physiological addiction? The next time you see some packaged, processed food, take a look at the ingredients list. If you can't pronounce some of the items in that list, the chances are very high that your body also doesn't

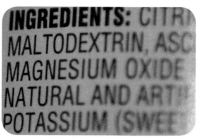

know what to do with these chemical ingredients. Eating these kinds of foods regularly might be thought of as a way of slowly embalming yourself. People often find it hard though, especially at the start, to consider as 'toxic' the foods they've loved and even *thought* were good for them.

> *"Toleration to poisons is merely a slow method of dying. Instead of seeing in the phenomena of toleration something to be sought after, it is something to seek to avoid the necessity for."*
> *--Herbert Shelton*

If you do have toxic processed foods like this in your house, it's a great idea to remove them immediately, if you can. (Only if they are yours of course – leave your housemates to their own food choices). You are also very likely malnourished and de-mineralised if you're eating such things, so your body constantly asks for more food to try to get some nutrients. Ironically, most people take that as a cue to eat even more of the 'only foods they know': de-mineralised, toxic junk food, which just clogs them up even more. Here are some of the top offenders in this area:

*processed starches (especially wheat): the opioids in wheat make it highly addictive and are the same kind of compounds found in morphine, used for pain relief. No wonder people feel 'comfort' from eating bread, cakes and cookies.

*refined sugars: we get hooked on blood-sugar highs and the brain chemicals released after consuming these nutrient-stripped sugars. Sugars are the body's natural fuel source - however, NOT refined sugars like white sugar, high-fructose corn syrup, etc. Dr. Norman Walker says in fact that, as they break down, the refined sugars create *alcohol* and acids in our systems (see his book *Become Younger*). Eating refined sugars also draws minerals out of your body.

*salt: 'standard' table salt is particularly damaging; it lines arteries, affects blood pressure and alters taste buds so that we cannot sense real flavours and hence, want more salt.

*coffee, black tea, colas: the caffeine stimulates us, runs down the adrenals, draws on our mineral reserves, stresses the liver.

*MSG, aspartame and other excitotoxins: all of these kinds of manu-factured 'flavour enhancers'/sweeteners and so on have been linked to ad-diction, obesity and cancers, plus they kill off brain neurons. MSG is often disguised in ingredient lists as 'natural flavours/seasoning/spices' etc.

In a sense, people could be said to be 'self-medicating' with these lacklustre foods. As raw food pioneer Dr. Ann Wigmore put it:

> "The food you eat can be either the safest and most powerful form of **medicine**, or the slowest form of **poison**."

Large amounts of refined sugars and simple carbs especially help people 'cope' with stress and discomfort by spacing out into sluggish, sleepy, stuffed and drugged states.

The fact that these foods are toxic and addictive is rarely, if ever, empha-sised in mainstream media, so most people never question the strength of their ties to these foods. It's often not simply these foods on their own that cause health issues for people – it's also the things they're processed or consumed *with*, such as pasteurised dairy products, factory-farmed meats, trans-fats and so on. If you find it hard to accept the idea that you might be physiologically *addicted* to foods like wheat, consider the fact that a smoker or alcoholic is not drawn to repeatedly use their 'drug' of choice from any kind of biological need. The body doesn't *need* cigarettes or alcohol. They are just addicted, in the same way as people eating refined sugar or drinking coffee.

There is *no* physiological benefit to you from consuming these things (in fact quite the opposite), yet you may feel repeatedly drawn to consume them. It is fundamentally an addiction, like any other. Yes, of course you need food to survive – however, you do not need to eat white sugar and wheat.

Not all foods are physiologically addictive. There are many natural, delicious and healthy options available. Fresh, living, raw foods like pears, broccoli and alfalfa, for example, are not usually linked to physical dependence. How many people do you see with a chronic kale addiction…? Switching over to a mainly raw food lifestyle can therefore make a huge difference for people in terms of liberating them from compulsive eating. Take away the toxic foods you're addicted to and you're half-way to freedom.

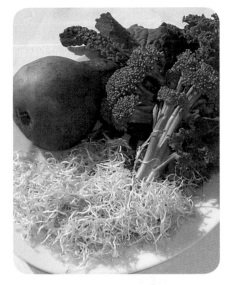

However, because raw foods simply don't 'tick the same boxes' in terms of addictive properties, if your diet has been highly processed until now, switching over to mainly or totally raw can feel quite harsh in the beginning. Raw foods don't create those drugged responses we have come to associate with comfort, reward or satisfaction. Suddenly the coping mechanisms we've been using to deal with discomfort for decades are *gone*. We might liken this to being on anti-depressant medication for 34 years, then suddenly removing it – it's quite a shock to the system. It's like having a safety net pulled out from under your feet or the smoky veil of processed food addiction grabbed down from before your eyes. Whichever way you look at it, the new landscape can seem pretty challenging. The 'comfort' element of eating is largely gone and we find ourselves, for perhaps the first time ever, actually feeling our emotional discomfort directly, rather than using food to self-medicate (shoving it down, finding 'comfort' and ignoring our feelings). As mentioned above, we might reach out for heavier raw foods like masses of nuts, seeds, gourmet raw pizza and so on to try to bridge that gap, yet even these don't sedate us in quite the same way as our old toxic food 'friends'.

Many people find this kind of shift very confrontational and are not sure how to handle the changes. They may feel impassioned about transforming their health, yet where do they find 'comfort' now, if food seems to no longer offer sanctuary?

It's easy to see here that the *psychological* aspects of food addiction certainly aren't guaranteed to vanish simply from going raw. For many, this part of the healing process can actually seem like a bigger issue to deal with than moving through the physical elements of withdrawal.

It's time for some major re-programming to release yourself from reliance on food as your 'safety net' and to start finding other things in your life that feel rewarding, satisfying and comforting to you, *beyond* the food. Remember, the menu of life is abundant with positive possibilities. This is where all the tips shared on the following pages come in - you can get AC-TIVE to turn things around for yourself. The fresh foods can help you to an extent, then *action* on the emotional/spiritual aspects is what will really help you to move on and heal on all levels.

Beware the Durian !

Are all raw foods non-addictive? I believe there are a few raw foods that can become physiologically addictive, among them cacao (raw chocolate), raw salt, raw wine, spices and...possibly durian fruit. These items are all raw, yet all seem to induce compulsive behaviour in some people. Cacao contains alkaloid compounds such as caffeine and theobromine, which can trigger addictions (some raw foodists even jokingly call raw chocolate 'cracao', in reference to its addictive properties). As for raw salt: you might be eating the greatest salt in the world, yet if you feel the need to use it in everything savoury you eat, it might be that you're dependent on it, rather than simply using it for flavouring/re-mineralisation. Raw wine contains alcohol of course and can hence be addictive. Spices tend to be powdered forms of certain plants, in concentrations you would not easily come across in nature. Spices are usually made by powdering down a large amount of a bark, root, or other plant matter, often heating them in the process. You might even have a spice *blend*. The concentrated intensity of the spice can throw the body a bit out of balance, as you are getting a much bigger 'hit' of this food than you'd naturally be able to easily get hold of if you were just foraging things to eat in the wild. This imbalance can distort taste buds, blocking your ability to sense when you've eaten enough and thereby encouraging eating in excess. As for durian (a large, spiky, 'stinky', yet incredible-tasting fruit from South-East Asia)...hmmm...the jury's out on this one I think, yet watching the frenzied enthusiasm with which many raw foodists eat this fruit, it would not be hard to imagine that it contains some physically addicting compounds.

I believe the vast majority of raw foods are not physiologically addictive; there are just a handful of things you might want to be vigilant about. Contrast this with the foods on offer in most *supermarkets* however and you'll find quite the opposite picture. The vast majority of foods sold in supermarkets are physiologically addictive, with just a few 'safe' areas outside the middle aisles, like the produce section. As my friend Kathy says, "The middle aisles will kill you".

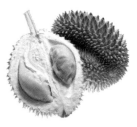

Durian Fruit

54

Are You Eating 'Raw' Yet...?

If not, I suggest that right now you start to include plenty of raw foods in your daily eating. Ideally, go for 50% raw today. At the very least, kick-start your journey by introducing one full plate of RAW foods daily. You might eat that raw plate *before* another meal or as a complete meal in itself.

How can you do this? It might mean that you make up a gorgeous fresh fruit salad for breakfast with perhaps banana, blueberries, peaches and grapes OR maybe it means that you eat a plate of delicious salad just before your usual evening meal. You could tuck in to a plate bursting with bright, flavourful veggies like crisp lettuce, spinach, cilantro, grated carrots and cucumbers, diced bell peppers, alfalfa sprouts and so on, covered with a vibrant dressing of avocado blended with lemon juice and dulse seaweed. Eating a simple raw salad before a more complex meal like traditional pasta with meatballs can really help with digestion; the raw veggies act like a kind of 'bullet-proof vest'.

Commit to this: every day, increase your raw intake until you reach at least 50% raw. Go by the *weight* of the foods rather than the volume; i.e., 50% of the *weight* of your food is raw, weighed against whatever else you are eating that day. You can achieve this comfortably within a few days. By starting to go raw as you read this book (if you haven't already) and steadily increasing your intake – up to 100% raw even, if you like – you'll be able to understand and benefit so much more from what is shared here. Remember that Appendices A and B contain lots of useful tips and recipes for healthy raw food eating.

We can ALL come up with any number of reasons why we feel we can't go raw at this point. It comes down to choice. Do you want to choose this for yourself? I know how it feels to face the path of raw foodism and feel daunted. I stood at that same crossroads in 2002 and had my choice to make. I chose a simple life of raw foods and natural healthcare. I may not still be here today if I had chosen a different path.

Eating more raw food doesn't have to be a big deal – this is, after all, about getting back to simplicity. Make it easy for yourself and just get started!

You may find following my 30-Day Raw Weight Loss Plan invaluable. It offers menu planners, recipes, daily instructional videos, community support, a fitness guide and much more. You can even choose between an all-raw plan or an 'Intermediate' option with cooked alternatives. See www.RevitaLivePlan.com for more details.

The Psychological Addiction and Cravings

In the Realisation and Transition stages especially, many people feel that they struggle with cravings for foods they no longer want to eat, or they hanker for excessive amounts of food. Why do cravings happen? Well, a big reason of course is that until you remove those foods that are highly *physiologically* addictive (like the processed starches and sugars) from the intake *completely*, they remain in your system and you stay addicted. Beyond the physiological addiction, however, there is much more to consider: the *psychological* aspects.

Most humans resist change strongly. We like things to feel easy and 'comfortable', rather than in flux. If your pattern has been to use those kinds of processed foods for comfort, you are naturally going to crave having those experiences again and to keep repeating them, rather than making shifts. You are craving familiarity and the sense of comfort that way of life brought for you. It can feel like a lonely road setting out on this healing path, especially if those around you don't support what you're doing. The cravings are a reflection of the associations in your head between food and comfort. Those associations have as much validity as you choose to give them. They can be restructured at any time, with new thought patterns, beliefs and choices. The more you keep moving into your new patterns, the less the old cravings will affect you. They fade with time and consistency. Again, the 'Guidance' section you'll find later in this book is absolutely packed with suggestions and exercises to help you handle cravings and create new patterns for yourself.

As previously noted, most of us start forming emotional associations with food from a very young age. Children are routinely given food to pacify them, cheer them up, reward them and so on. This creates strong psychological bonds between our feelings and our food. Many children are coerced into eating when they're not hungry, finishing meals 'to make Mummy happy' and so on. Eating thus becomes a way of getting approval and finding comfort and happiness. It is mostly a false kind of happiness though, when examined more closely. Far from bringing genuine joy, the child gets hooked into life-long patterns of 'using' foods that are potentially damaging. There is a genuine joy in life far sweeter than any candy bar, which we can all access at any moment simply by choosing to pay attention to our true feelings and coming into alignment with what is 'natural', i.e., nature.

If children grow up understanding that food is a way to get approval and attention, they may develop control patterns around eating as a way to try to control their environment. Many children quietly feel unseen and unaccepted by their caregivers, receiving little 'mirroring' for their true selves. Healthy mirroring means that someone is there for the child, reflects an accurate image of who they really are, acknowledges their point of view and gives them un-

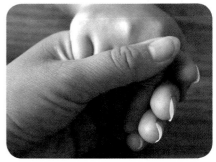

conditional love. However, disturbed communication patterns like blaming and shaming from critical and unaffectionate adults can leave children feeling lonely. Children themselves are often not even conscious of exactly what is happening, they only know that they don't feel good. As a result, they may engage in other-than-optimal eating habits as one way to try to get some sense of control of *something* – in this case, their body – in an environment that feels hostile and unloving. Just like all of us, children are looking for love and acceptance at all times. When they don't receive this directly from their caregivers, they may turn to food, drugs, graffiti, self-mutilation, computers, alcohol, gambling or any number of other diversions from their frustrations. They might restrict or grossly over-use

Life Beyond the Loop

*I no longer get cravings for cooked/processed foods. They don't even LOOK like food to me – they look toxic. Why would I put something into my body that looks toxic to me? It was quite a journey to get to this point, though. I experienced some intense cravings/bingeing with cooked foods at the start of my raw journey, mainly because I didn't cut out refined sugars and starches **completely**.*

*I recall sitting with a friend who'd stopped eating refined sugars and was helping me do the same. We were at a café and the waiter served us complimentary foil-wrapped chocolates with our tea. I felt immensely frustrated, as I really wanted to eat them and so much of my attention was focused on them. I looked at my friend sitting calmly and asked her if she wasn't frustrated too, seeing the chocolates and not eating them. She gently smiled and said, 'No, I look and see they have pretty pictures on the wrapper...I don't desire to eat them'. At that point, her perspective seemed so far away from mine that I almost couldn't imagine ever feeling that way towards these blocks of processed dairy/sugars/cocoa. These days, however, I don't feel any effort in avoiding my old Trigger foods (like doughnuts, for example), as they simply don't interest me anymore and are so far from the spectrum of foods I now choose. If that sounds like something you'd like to experience too, just keep on reading and **taking action**.*

foods as a subtle form of 'rebellion', which unfortunately usually further depletes their own health and well-being.

It is common to find people still acting out these self-destructive patterns decades later. For example, you might see a fifty-year-old woman still diving for the ice cream tub every time she feels hurt. Once embedded, these patterns can be tough to shift. Indeed, for some people, controlling the flow of food that goes into their body might feel like one of the only things they really have control over. They have given so much of their power and joy away to activities and thought patterns that essentially keep them miserable. Food seems like the only true constant ally, the silent crutch to lean on, the escape hatch into oblivion...

Resistance

Another key reason people experience cravings is because they are in a state of resistance towards certain foods and behaviours. Realise that *what we resist persists*. When you make something into a forbidden food for yourself and speak in terms of being 'not able' or 'not *allowed*' to eat certain things, you are approaching the situation from a weakened, rather than empowered standpoint. Perhaps you also try to make rules for yourself like 'I only eat pizza once a week' or ultimatums like 'this is THE last time I'm going to eat this, EVER'. This kind of thinking can easily lead to rebellion. After withholding from the 'banned' foods for a while, we often pitch full-force into compulsive overeating sessions. Creating a sense of restriction around your food choices can lead to some hefty backlashes, especially from the 'child' inside, who does not want to be told what to do. If this sounds like you, try this little turnaround: consider that rather than living with restrictions, you are making wonderful, positive new lifestyle choices for yourself - the Guidance section (pgs. 162-216) is packed with tips to support your transformation.

No-one is saying that you CAN'T eat this or SHOULDN'T eat that. It is about getting informed about the effect foods really have on you and then making *choices* from there, for yourself.

Can you see that if there is nothing you are 'denying' yourself, there would be nothing to feel a craving for? The truth is, since everything is available to you to choose (as it is), then what you put into your mouth is simply a matter of your own *choice*. If you are thinking about your food choices from an empowered place where you know that, for example, you *could* eat bread if you wanted to, you may find that you just don't want to - a perspective that seems a lot more gentle than restricted thinking such as 'I'm *not* allowed to eat this bread', leading to compulsive outbreaks. Drop the restrictions in your head, re-frame your thinking, accept that you can eat anything you want and you may find that suddenly...many of those cravings vanish. There is simply nothing to resist anymore.

If you find a lot of your energy going towards *worrying* about how you're going to resist certain foods, consider this: you are giving your power away to that very thing you're resisting. Move your focus elsewhere - distract yourself with something that delights you. Bring your power back to positive creations in your life, rather than...doughnuts ;)

In your Transition, you might also find that if you soften into a craving - let's say it's rice cakes, for example – and enjoy eating that food for a few days, you discover that the energy and interest then dissipates and you feel completely 'done' with that craving. Rather than resisting, you made it OK for yourself and went with it. The energy to eat rice cakes is then satisfied and released.

Tracking Your Course Away from Cravings

I believe the easiest healing path we can take for ourselves is to get educated about the impact of different foods, create a vision of where we would LOVE to be in terms of our health (as we'll be doing in this book), marry this with appropriate food intake and head out in the direction of that vision. You then have a sense of where you're going with this and can begin setting aside the main 'nasties', as you enjoy the journey. Sure, you may still get cravings and you may find that you don't put down all the toxic foods *completely*, overnight. Yet underlying your behaviour, you are conscious of what those foods are likely doing to you. It is not that you are uninformed, you are just taking the journey more slowly towards your destination of happy, healthy Maintenance, forgiving any 'blips' along the way. Viewed in this way, cravings don't need to be a drama – they are just small obstacles along the journey. Cravings come and go and in every moment you are free to decide how you respond to them.

I came to understand something about my own patterns with cravings while on this journey that really helped me to **stop compulsive eating**. I came to accept that pretty much whatever I looked at, I wanted to eat (aside from things I didn't like, such as seafood). If it was within my view, I wanted to eat it, regardless of whether I was hungry or not. I just wanted to eat anything I laid my eyes on – it was like an endless craving to fill, fill, fill myself. At that time, as a rampant binge-eating toxic food consumer, the impact I was having on my health every time I acted on that urge to eat was far more damaging than as a raw food eater. However, the compulsion doesn't simply vanish just from going raw. After I went raw, it was still there. It didn't matter which **raw** foods I was looking at or what time of day it was, I wanted to eat. Even as a 100% raw food eater, the spectrum of things I was attracted to had shifted completely, yet the wild *compulsion* remained to eat all that I could. After a while I came to understand this pattern and how destructive and all-pervasive it was for me. I came to see that it was basically inevitable that if I looked at food, I wanted to eat it. When I saw that clearly, it really helped me relax and even laugh at the absurdity of it.

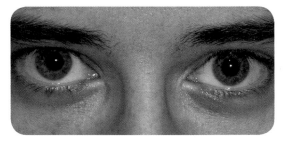

With time I learned to examine the many emotional/spiritual tangles underlying that pattern and to stop acting out on every impulse. I accepted the pattern thus far for what it was and learned to breathe deeply into each incident and let go, rather than acting out. I found too that the longer I was on a raw path, the more cleansing my body experienced and hence the less food it asked for. The demands for food just naturally declined and the patterns have changed now. I may still look at things and think, 'wow, that looks yummy', yet it doesn't mean I want to eat it right then. Mindless *instant gratification* like that just doesn't feel like a healthy or happy choice to me anymore. I want to make choices that better support my health and well-being in the long run, rather than compulsively munching.

Diets Don't Work

Doctors, nutritionists, friends and family may all urge us to use them; magazines may offer new 'diets' every week; we may obsess over various 'miracle' plans; yet almost without exception, *diets* do not produce satisfactory and permanent results. Why do dieters often lose some weight, only to gain it all back again, plus more, when the diet ends? Quite simply, mainstream diets only address the 'weight problem' and ignore the crucial component of addiction/emotional attachment. The focus is often confined to some isolated aspect of nutrition, such as calorie counting, with the dieter directed to put attention exclusively on that, rather than considering the broader picture.

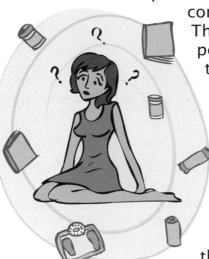

There is also little to no understanding of the **detox** process that is inevitable when anyone starts to eat less. Most people are in a constant state of *intoxifying* themselves with food and drink. They never give their bodies a break to release anything. As a result of this, the average person in Western societies is now said to gain one pound a year in weight. If, however, they break up the 'intoxifying' process by eating less or at least eating *differently* with a diet, their cells will finally get a chance to 'exhale' and they will go into detox. This detox process can feel very unpleasant. It is no different in principle to a heroin addict coming off their drug. Processed foods like white sugar and standard flour are HIGHLY addictive substances, yet this relationship is not widely understood or accepted in society. So people go on diet regimes that offer little support for their experiences and often end up feeling confused, deprived and miserable.

If you struggle to understand that foods like wheat and sugar are highly addictive, consider this: you may hear someone who is sixty pounds overweight saying that they need to eat something to give them energy. Logically, of course, this makes *no* sense. They are obviously already carrying ample stores of extra energy in their body – sixty pounds of it. Yet they still feel that they 'need' more food for energy. The reality is, they don't need it for energy – they have become physically addicted to the food they eat (aside from the fact that they're also almost certainly malnourished from these poor food choices). They are using this food for emotional reasons and to STOP the pains of detox that begin as soon as they stop consuming their regular flow of toxins. This is no different from a cigarette smoker who might feel the 'need' for a cigarette, when clearly there is no physiological *need* for someone to smoke tobacco; they are simply addicted. For all these reasons and more, it is tough for anyone to lose weight healthily and permanently with mainstream dieting.

When dieting, people may also feel very weak, as they are getting fewer calories and not necessarily from foods that nourish them well. Toxins are pouring into their system from eating less (released from fat storage, to be eliminated), yet many do no colon cleansing (enemas, colonics, etc.) to help facilitate the release of that waste. On top of that, they are quite likely feeling miserable and 'restricted' with the diet plan. This certainly doesn't seem like an optimal scenario.

This kind of dieting pattern rarely seems to *genuinely* help empower people into a new way of life. We often go 'on' diets so that we can go 'off' them again once we have reached a particular target weight. Then we revert back to old patterns, somehow expecting things to work out differently this time. It is a simple fact that repeatedly engaging in the same behaviour brings the same results.

When viewed from the outside like this, it is clear that this standard dieting pattern is not rational, yet this is how millions of people try repeatedly to manage their perceived 'weight problem'. Many diets are doomed from the start, as they do not *completely* exclude the most common toxic 'Trigger' foods for compulsive eating, like wheat and sugar, so the cycle of craving is never broken. Instead, the dieter

> ## Are you stuck in the 'dieting trap'?
>
> Do any of these patterns below sound familiar?
>
> *counting your calories
> *obsessing about weighing yourself
> *repeatedly making statements like 'I'll start going raw on Monday...'
> *feeling like you're restricting yourself
> *comparing yourself to others and wishing you were thinner
>
> If so, please recognise this pattern as the 'dieting mentality' of an outdated paradigm, which there is no need to adhere to. Enjoying a raw food lifestyle can be about making positive, healthy, uplifting choices EVERY day – not just for a couple of weeks or until we lose the weight or go 'off' our plan.
> Living foods are for life, not just for weight loss!

remains hooked enough on limited quantities of these 'drugs' to experience a deep sense of deprivation during the diet, until they come 'off' the diet merry-go-round again. Sooner or later, bingeing usually resumes. From start to finish, this whole 'dieting' pattern tends to feel very unpleasant for the one having the experience. Feeling persistently uncomfortable is not a logical pathway to vibrant, sustainable health.

In contrast, a clear benefit of the way of eating shared in *this* book is that all toxic Trigger foods are ideally *completely* omitted with a high-raw lifestyle, plus you'll find here many supportive tools for your emotional, mental, social and spiritual transformation. Initially, at the physical level, it's what you consistently *don't* eat that kick–starts your fullest healing. Some people might lose weight with a standard diet, yet they don't feel that healthy or look very vibrant. They may still get ill, gain weight back and live with degenerative diseases. They have not omitted the most toxic food groups and they don't *feel* good about the process.

In contrast, a raw food lifestyle is so healing because you leave out everything *except* raw (vegan) options. The body finally gets a chance to clear out old debris, then rebuilds, using these supportive foods. It's a completely different approach to standard dieting. Yes, there are still likely to be moments of discomfort going raw, especially as you explore the detox processes. The huge difference here, however, lies in the *outcome*, which can bring not just healthy, rapid, sustainable weight loss, but healing transformation on so many levels.

Diets also tend to keep food addicts obsessed with food, as they're often so complicated that people become very preoccupied with them. Some also involve dangerously low calorie intakes that provide inadequate nutrition and leave the body in a state of starvation, triggering the *storage* rather than loss of fat.

Dieting can feel lonely if there is no support system, which is another reason why many people end up slipping in and out of countless diets. Even those diet clubs that DO offer a support system of some kind – like weekly meetings – often do not address any of the underlying emotional issues, so the chances of sustained transformation are still compromised. (Info on where to find a *raw* support system is provided in the 'Sharing Circles' section of the Guidance chapter, plus the 'Resources' section, both later in this book.)

Many dieters end up blaming themselves when they don't see desired results; they view the experience as a personal failure, adding more shame to an already battered self-image. Mainstream diets don't address excess weight as a *symptom* of food addictions, which can themselves be seen as symptoms of a larger spiritual malady. Most people don't realise, therefore, that standard diets are set up to 'fail', by treating the *symptom* and not the core condition. When the addiction and imbalanced emotional connection are properly addressed, as with the lifestyle outlined in this book, the symptoms, like excess weight, take care of themselves.

The same pattern is seen with exercise regimes that people obsess over as 'miracle' weight-loss cures. Sustainable results are rarely seen, as this is another approach that ignores the underlying condition and only addresses the weight issue. Lack of information about food addiction and emotional issues leaves many blundering about in cycles of self-disgust and crash-dieting/exercise plans, with no healthy strategy for releasing these patterns. If this all sounds unpleasantly familiar, those days are over. Now is the time to stop dieting: choose transformation with a healthy raw lifestyle and start really living...

Get Perspective

'Waste not, want not'...? No need, there's always the compost...

If you struggle with the habit of wanting to 'not waste' any food and find, as a result, that you often end up eating more than you'd ideally like to, try to view this from a broader perspective. One way or another, everything returns to the Earth. Consider the fact that there is SO much food in the world and it is not *your* personal responsibility to eat it. Mother Earth produces food continuously, regardless of whether or not *you* are going to eat it. Those foods that are neither harvested nor consumed simply return to the Earth. You may choose to 'take responsibility' for a portion of the foods produced by purchasing them, but it doesn't mean that even these foods **must** be con-

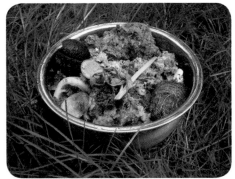

sumed by you. It is of no ultimate consequence whether those foods return to the Earth after passing through your body or by going directly in the compost bin. What seems more important, is the level of self-respect and self-love we demonstrate by not filling our bodies with unwanted, excess food. Better in the waste than *on* the waist!

Try to eat with love, intention and consciousness, treating your body as a 'temple', rather than a waste disposal unit. Ensure that EVERY thing you take into your body is something you feel great about. Avoid emptying a plate just to empty it. If it helps you, try eating each meal with the kind of reverence and enjoyment you might expect to feel if this was to be the last meal you ever eat. Wouldn't you choose the finest things for yourself and savour every mouthful? Why not choose to eat that way *all* the time, eating things you feel great about rather than sloppy leftovers and wilted greens?

If you find yourself with leftovers after a meal, resist temptations to eat them all immediately and instead store them for some alternative use, even freezing them if necessary. Throwing out food tends to be very confrontational for food addicts. However, if something would be better given back to the Earth, *do* it – it is far preferable to 'waste' a small quantity of unwanted food than fill your body with un-needed material. Try it sometime, as an experience, if you're not used to throwing leftovers away. How does it feel? New? Empowering? Scary? Irritating? Value your body and your recovery more than some leftover food.

> ### Eating with Intention
> A wonderful gift you can give yourself daily is to eat with loving intention. Accompany each meal with thoughts such as:
>
> "It is my intention that this food is optimally assimilated by my body. This meal helps me feel nourished, balanced and healthy. I enjoy this meal with love and gratitude."

'But it costs money...'

If, on close examination, the 'honest' reason you tell yourself that you want to eat something is because you or someone else paid *money* for it, consider the fact that you're seemingly more concerned about the health of your wallet than your body. Do you really want to take excess foods into your body just because you *bought* them? In the end, would you rather have your bank account a little out of balance, or your *body*...? If your budget is a concern, I

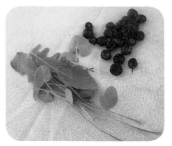

suggest going out and foraging for free, fresh, vibrant berries, fruits, shoots and greens, straight from nature, plus sprouting and growing your own produce.

You may not feel able to implement these ideas around 'waste' immediately. Indeed, it might take many years before you feel genuinely willing and able to consistently not eat leftovers. Everyone's process is different, so just take things at a pace *you* feel comfortable with - simply being *aware* of these ideas for now is a good start. You can always re-visit these suggestions further down the line...

Also, from the long-term perspective, consider viewing eating raw as an amazing and solid investment in your health and longevity, plus the health of the whole planet. It might seem expensive to eat organic, for example, yet in the long term you will have fewer health issues to deal with as a result of your choices, which means fewer potential medical costs further down the line, plus a healthier life for yourself and the planet. Eating organic helps build a truly healthy economy. In our 'ADD' (Attention Deficit Disorder) cultures, so many people seem to focus on immediate satisfaction. People compromise their long-term health in preference for instant gratification by, for example, biting into a processed, packaged product to which they are addicted, rather than sourcing and preparing fresh organic foods. If you want

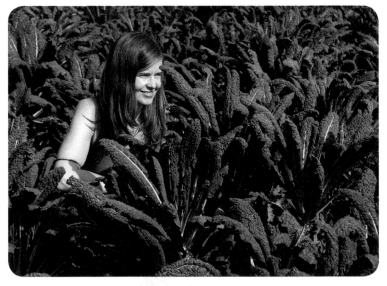

to eat those kinds of processed foods and are sincerely enjoying that way of life, then that is your choice. If you want to focus more on the bigger perspective and embrace a healthier way of living and eating for **all** concerned, then the guidance shared here is designed to give you inspiration and tools for that lifestyle.

Living with 'Toxic' Emotional Attachment to Food – How Does it Feel?

There are many different ways that someone's emotional connection with food may manifest, from the mild and innocuous to the extreme and highly detrimental. As we've seen, some people experience happy and fulfilling emotional connections with their food – such as the 'Happy Humans' and those in 'Maintenance'. Others have a much more toxic-feeling relationship with food. For example, some people get into patterns of restriction and control around food (an extreme example being anorexia), others get into binge/purge patterns, some may 'use' food to manipulate others such as their children and so on. Even someone with a high-raw lifestyle may feel toxic if they still attach feelings like guilt, shame and stress to their food intake. This keeps them in an acid, toxic state – again, simply being raw isn't *the* answer to emotional food issues. These 'toxic' emotional connections seem a far cry from the simplistic, more primal connection with food that we see in wild animals or 'Animalistic Humans'.

While there are many ways in which emotional connections with food may be expressed, in my view by *far* the most common manifestation of this in our societies is overeating. This is therefore the main form of emotional attachment we'll focus on here. Please do understand though that by choosing to focus on the *positive* aspects of our relationship with food, eating with loving intention and allowing healing to unfold, we can *all* reach a balanced place of Maintenance, regardless of where we are coming from - bulimics, overeaters, controlling mothers and more.

'I Was Fine, Until I Started Eating Raw...'

Paradoxically, some may feel that they never actually had compulsive issues around food *until* they started to eat raw and now their eating feels a bit 'out of control' to them. This pattern tends to crop up for those who dive into being 100% or very high raw, very quickly. Suddenly putting down the foods with which we've been 'self-medicating' for years and instead facing our emotions head-on can feel very intense, triggering bingeing extremes. To me, this bingeing behaviour also seems to reflect an issue of restriction. The 'inner child' does not enjoy what it senses as a feeling of restriction/deprivation and being told what to do. The result is rebellion, with a passionate drive to overeat on whatever **does** seem to be acceptable and accessible, as this seems like the only outlet for expression in a restricted framework where, in terms of choices, people can feel boxed into a corner. It's very easy to see how this kind of compulsive behaviour emerges.

Very often, it is people on the margins of society who feel drawn towards eating raw. These 'extremists' may find that being raw stirs up lots of issues inside them and one result of this is swinging between eating styles. However, repeatedly bingeing or 'yo-yoing' between being very high/totally raw and eating junk/cooked/processed foods can both be quite damaging physically, as well as draining and disturbing emotionally.

If you find yourself with a surprising compulsion to overeat within the raw food boundaries you've chosen, OR you're swinging wildly from raw to 'junk' extremes, you'll do well to relax, breathe deeply and maybe take a step back from putting so many sudden pressures on yourself about what and how you eat. I would *far* prefer to see someone 80% raw, relaxed, happy and eating moderate amounts than 100% raw and barely holding themselves together, bingeing and feeling awful. Yes, going raw is new territory for most of us. However, with loving attention and understanding, we can lighten up the journey; it does not have to feel like a hostile and difficult terrain.

Life as An Overeater - How Did I Get There?

"Addiction: any process used to avoid or take away intolerable reality."
--Pia Mellody

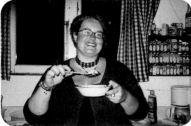

How does someone (like me) end up weighing 300 pounds? Well, for me, it was mainly the result of **compulsive overeating** – a highly destructive, addicted, emotional connection with food. I was using food as my escape hatch from my own 'intolerable reality'. I was completely obsessed with eating. If I was awake, I was most likely either eating or thinking about food. Life for me was like a series of opportunities to eat. I was definitely in the 'Passive Human' category during my obese years (perhaps I fell more into the 'Happy Human' category at the very start of my overeating journey – it rapidly descended into an uncomfortable relationship though.)

Leading self-help writer Charles L. Whitfield describes eating disorders such as compulsive overeating as 'A recurring pattern...usually used unconsciously to avoid authentic relationship with self or others'. The overeater, like all addicts, is out of touch with his or her true self and using food to try to fill the aching gap within.

It is my impression that, in our societies, overeating is experienced by so many people and yet recognised by very few. It seems rather ironic that this condition receives so little recognition, seeing as one of the common results – overweight or obesity – is so *visible* and prevalent. Yet it's as though we have a cultural blind spot for the truth about this issue. Usually, those with overweight or obesity issues will receive the message from doctors/society in general to 'just eat less and exercise more. Use your willpower, go on a diet'. There is little to no recognition given to emotional health or anything beyond the cold, hard, physical equation of 'calories in, calories out'.

*The physically addictive nature of modern foods is glossed over.
*The emotional turmoil that may be underlying the obesity is ignored.
*The reality that recovery takes knowledge + willINGNESS rather than
  willPOWER is overlooked.

As these aspects are so rarely openly discussed, people dealing with food addictions often remain stuck in patterns that no longer serve them, feeling miserable and isolated. They do not yet have access to the information or tools to help them move out of their rut. These people would mostly be found in our categories of Passive Human and Realisation. Some might even fluctuate between Realisation and Transition stages. Many will repeatedly try out different diets, only to regain any weight lost and remain feeling stuck and miserable.

The phrase 'you are what you eat' rarely seems to be taken literally. There is an apparent *large* disconnect in understanding the relationship between what we consume and the health of our bodies. (Just look at most foods served in hospitals for example.) We are so indoctrinated into believing that certain foods are 'good for us' – or at least harmless – plus we're so addicted to these toxic creations that we mostly overlook the reality that many people are destroying themselves with these foods. Very few people seem to want to look beyond the status quo, acknowledge what is really happening and make shifts. After all, everyone else in society seems to eat that way; doctors frequently insist that health has

> ## Avoiding Exposure
>
> *As a morbidly obese person, one of my primary missions at all times was to not draw attention to myself - rather ironic, given my size. I lived in fear of comments about my weight. I was terrified of the word 'fat' – I literally felt unable to say or hear it. As far as I was concerned, my weight was strictly taboo. In my obese body, I avoided contact with anyone I thought might make comments and tried not to aggravate anybody, as my weight seemed an easy point to joke about if someone was angry with me.*
>
> *I especially avoided contact with children, terrified of their potentially painful honesty. I feel sad about this now, but at the time I saw it as an essential part of my 'defences'. One encounter with a little girl who asked me point-blank, 'Why is your belly so big?' was enough to convince me that kids were a serious 'threat' to my bubble of denial...*
>
> *Living with all this fear, I developed many co-dependent tendencies. I desperately wanted acceptance from everybody and would over-extend myself in all directions, trying to people-please. It was as though I thought that if I was nice enough to everyone, they wouldn't make fun of me and I'd be ok. I was always 'on guard' in any social situation for potential criticism and if I didn't hear any, it felt like I'd 'got away', unharmed. If anything **was** said, I'd pretend to ignore it in public, then in private go over and over it in my head, feeling awful about it. It was an emotionally exhausting way to live and it's a great relief to be free of those concerns and patterns now.*

nothing to do with food intake; the unhealthy foods are usually the cheapest and most available; plus people feel 'too busy' to focus much on their nutrition, so they just go with the flow and eat the processed foods in restaurants and from supermarket shelves.

Many food addicts go through life feeling unworthy, inadequate and afraid. Their lives might feel unmanageable, lost in endless broken promises of 'I'm only going to have one', 'I'm *never* going to eat that again' or 'this time it will work'. We may even use our eating (unconsciously) as a kind of self-defeating control mechanism against a parent or spouse. We often compare ourselves to other people or to some 'perfect' ideal of ourselves. There is a wonderful phrase that for me really sums up how I felt as a food addict, before my transformation:

'When my inside looked at your outside,
I overate.'

We may judge ourselves by how we imagine other people to be and long desperately to feel as good as we *assume* they do.

Overeaters also commonly disconnect and isolate themselves, especially those who've become obese. Physical contact can become awkward and minimal. The obese person experiences little intimacy and often low or no sexual activity. Obese people may feel self-disgust and great shame about their physical appearance and might try to hide under baggy clothes, unwilling or unable to participate in activities such as swimming, for example, where they feel over-exposed. It's also harder to keep larger bodies clean and free from infection, so obese people may carry unpleasant body odours more frequently than others, which can contribute to ostracising.

The psychological and emotional consequences of living in such a greatly overburdened body can feel very draining, often resulting in depression, low self-esteem, self-pity and much anxiety. For many obese overeaters, isolation becomes a way of life.

Overeaters repeatedly turn to food as a crutch to try to help them feel happier. They are desperate to feel happy, yet the tool they are picking up – food – ironically leaves them stuck in circles of addiction, irrational thinking and self-defeating behaviour. We can see how, for many overweight overeaters, isolation and introversion become a way of life.

Tell-Tale Signs of An Overeater...

How can *you* know if you are an overeater or not? Well, ultimately, it's really up to you to decide whether you choose to identify yourself that way. In this section I'll give some pointers about the typical behaviour and classic thought patterns of those who eat compulsively and to excess. You can read it over, see if you 'tick any boxes' and decide for yourself.

Do Any of These Sound Familiar?
*I am overweight or obese.
(Many overeaters are either overweight or obese. *However* – not **all** overeaters carry signs of their addiction so visibly. Some may be a standard weight for their size, yet still have compulsive issues with food.)

*A great deal of my time and energy is directed towards food. I find it difficult to be present with people or concentrate on activities because my thoughts are preoccupied with food.

*I eat in secret, binge-eat, fluctuate between bingeing and deprivation, eat when I'm not hungry, hide food wrappers, am dishonest about what I've eaten, find I start eating and feel like I 'just can't stop' and so on.

*I eat moderately in front of others, then 'make up for it' in private with binges, especially on refined sugars and processed starches: ice cream, cakes, cookies, chips, etc.

*I feel compelled to eat everything available – I do not want to 'waste' anything, so I eat everything on my plate, often picking scraps/leftovers from fellow diners too.

*I go to sleep excited to wake up the next day so that I can eat again. I awake to thoughts of what I'm going to eat that day. Food seems to be the highlight of my days and yet ironically, I often feel terrible after eating.

*When I eat, my mood changes perceptibly – I use food for comfort, to pacify myself, deal with stress, reward myself, celebrate and so on. During and afterwards, I might feel guilt, shame, remorse, fear, self-disgust and more.

*I live in a crazy internal landscape where an obsession with slimness and body image exists in constant battle with the compulsion to eat. I typically look for a solution in endless cycles of dieting and weigh myself frequently.

*I might be very 'particular' and rigid, almost ritualistic, about the circumstances in which I want to eat. I may get upset and angry if the situation doesn't seem to fit my ideal.

(This is not to be confused with having simple preferences, such as blessing food before eating. The pattern described above tends to be more specific and uncompromising, indicating a strong attachment to eating habits.)

I remember when I first looked over a similar list to this, I could identify with almost every characteristic of overeating listed. Yet I thought little of it. I really didn't realise that this kind of relationship with food might be considered imbalanced.

It was only when I asked my partner at that time if he identified with these traits and discovered that he answered 'no' to almost every item that the strangeness of my own behaviour finally struck me. Other people didn't do these things... This came as a surprise to me and I tried to imagine how different their relationship must be to food. To not spend a large portion of the day thinking about food (what, when and how to eat next); feeling able to leave food on the plate if full or to refuse food if not hungry; being able to keep and eat a bar of chocolate over a number of days, rather than wolfing the whole thing down in seconds – how different life would be if I were to behave like that.

"For the overeater, one compulsive bite of food is too many and a thousand is never enough."
--'Overeaters Anonymous' saying

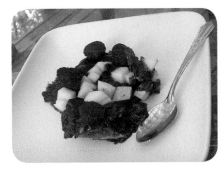

You cannot fill an aching spiritual chasm with something physical. With hindsight, the fact that I didn't even realise that my relationship with food was odd speaks volumes to me about how overeating is so glossed-over and even 'mainstream' in our societies. Whereas known alcoholics are unlikely to find people offering them drinks, food is something that people commonly share with others, obese overeaters included. As I have said, I consider addiction to highly processed foods and overeating to be among the most common addictions in the modern world. It's so common in fact that it's barely seen as unusual or even acknowledged. Plus, there is also the chance that if the eating pattern of one person in a community is called into question, others might fear (consciously or subconsciously) that the spotlight will be turned on their own eating patterns and they therefore avoid the topic completely.

Let's take a closer look at compulsion:

Com.pul.sion n.

"An irresistible impulse to act, regardless of the rationality of the motivation" (Definition from www.dictionary.com)

Compulsive behaviour is not logical – it is something we do *in spite of ourselves*, our willpower or any good intentions we may have. For food addicts,

The Absurd Dance of Compulsion

Before I started to work on my emotional transformation, my compulsive behaviour with food was quite remarkable. For example, before Christmas in Iceland (where I used to live), stores usually put out cookies, cakes and candy for customers to enjoy. I would find myself cycling all over the city, from store to store, just to eat the treats on offer. I didn't actually need anything in the stores, yet in the midst of a cold Icelandic winter, I was willing to bicycle through ice and snow for hours just to eat 'treats'. Similarly, I used to love going to the bank in Iceland, as they give free hot chocolate. Whenever my partner at the time would say he was going to the bank, I'd excitedly ask, 'Can I come?', to his bemusement. I was in the grip of compulsion and food was my focus.

My compulsive behaviour with food probably reached its peak of insanity when I began working in a mainstream café where the staff were permitted to eat whatever they wanted, whenever they wanted...an overeater's paradise and worst nightmare, rolled into one. Every day I worked there, I ate much more than I physically needed to, time and time again finding myself eating things that caused me physical pain and emotional turmoil. Bread, ice cream, cakes, chips...

For weeks at a time I'd battle my compulsion to overeat, stuffing lump after lump of cake into my mouth. At times, my willpower to stop would win over and I'd be able to halt the madness for some days or even weeks. Overall, however, I was really out of balance. Looking back, I can see how I treated my body like a waste disposal system. I had no sense of honouring my self or making healthy choices about what I consumed. I couldn't bear to see food 'go to waste', so on top of my own multiple meals, I would gobble down leftovers from customers' plates. It seems insane now, but that was my reality then.

I was actually very ill with a candida overgrowth at that point and ironically, though I'd taken myself off all fruit 'for health reasons', I was simultaneously filling myself compulsively with toxic refined sugars. Such is the absurd 'logic' of compulsion. I felt very ashamed, hiding my binges from co-workers and it took me a long time to find the courage to even tell my partner about what I was doing.

this applies not only to what and how much we eat, but also the ways in which we try to control our food – for example, eating in secret or when we are not hungry, bingeing then purging or alternating between overeating and starvation.

Many develop obesity and other serious health issues as a physical result of overloading daily with excessive amounts of food. They simply do not receive the message that their obesity is actually a *symptom* of a compulsive addiction, which is itself a symptom of a bigger spiritual malady. Nor do they realise that help is available, through books like this and support groups. The excess weight is not the issue in and of itself. Many overeaters spend huge amounts of money, time and energy attempting to control what is perceived as merely a 'weight problem'. From diets to shots to surgery to slimming pills, we've tried it all, only to find that somehow we are still overweight, still miserable and still drawn compulsively to overeat.

It is important to understand too that *many of our perceived issues arise **from** our overeating* and not the other way around. You may hear people say, for example, that they reach out for food and overeat *because* they feel 'so unhappy, fat, stressed and want comfort food' or '*because* my partner is so mean to me' and so on. However, our overeating isn't *caused* by someone else's behaviour towards us, or the fact that we are overweight. There is also

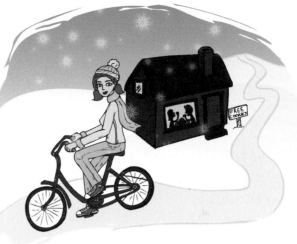

no need to try to justify compulsions. Overeating is simply a choice. Making food our 'ally' and compulsively eating large amounts is a pattern that some people play out again and again. This can in turn lead to myriad 'issues' in our lives. It often ends up as a vicious circle, yet we *can* step outside that circle by examining our behaviour and consciously starting to make different choices.

People may therefore go into personal transformation work not because they want to stop having their substance of choice, but because *they want to stop feeling unhappy about their choices.* As food addicts, if we could go into a kind of recovery where 'suffering' ceased and we could happily continue eating all we wanted, I'm sure the vast majority of us would jump at the chance. It is not so much that we want to stop *eating*, it is just that we don't want to be in pain anymore – we want to feel great.

An Addiction Like Any Other

Addiction is addiction, only the substances/activities differ. We can use or abuse *anything* as our escape hatch. Toxic foods just happened to suit me. Overeaters are addicts like any others. Just like an alcoholic might desperately seek out the next drink, overeaters may take food secretly, lie, hide food from others and so on. The overeaters' substance of choice also happens to be plentiful, legal and cheap in our societies. Thus, very little can get in the way of an overeater on a mission to eat. They may be able to keep other addictive substances in their home and have no issues with them whatsoever, like alcohol for example. Yet if there is a *single* chocolate in the house, it seems nothing will stop them from finding and eating it. Such is the nature of compulsive addiction. For those who feel they've never had this kind of relationship with food (or anything else), such behaviour might seem distinctly odd.

Most of us reading this book live in societies where there is the illusion of widespread abundance. We don't reside in tiny mountain villages in Bhutan, for example, living simply from the land. In our societies we are surrounded by potential distractions; there are so many different things for us to use or abuse – cigarettes, alcohol, food, prescription drugs, etc. We are, for the most part, far from a situation where we're looking to meet our basic needs. We also tend to be pretty disconnected from nature and a simple, constant link with Spirit. This can leave us with an aching, intangible gap within. We feel other–than–wonderful and try to fill this internal hole. Many people pick up food as their number-one 'drug of choice' to try to fill that empty space inside. Food is an 'easy' choice in this regard, being readily available, cheap and even ENCOURAGED socially, as well as massively promoted through advertising.

In contrast to, for example, a substance like alcohol, which we do not need to survive but can become addicted to, food is something we cannot normally live without (a few yogis/breatharians excepted). This makes food addiction much more common and even 'mainstreamed' in places, plus tends to encourage the feeling that it's tougher to break food addiction than other addictions. There is an anecdotal saying among Overeaters Anonymous (OA) members: "When you are addicted to drugs you put the tiger in the cage to recover; when you are addicted to food you put the tiger in the cage, but take it out three times a day for a walk."

Personally, I struggled at first to accept that I'd become addicted to something I need to survive. Whereas I could clearly understand someone being addicted to alcohol, smoking, drugs, work, gambling and so on, it was a different thing altogether for me to comprehend that I had developed an unhealthy dependence on *food* as my mood-altering substance of choice.

However, I did not clearly see the distinction then between life-supporting, natural and nourishing *raw foods* and toxic, chemical, addictive junk foods. I merely thought 'how can food be addictive?', without considering the composition or physiological effects of the *junk* that made up the bulk of my intake. If we learn to differentiate and stop thinking of those things as 'food' at all, it can change the way we see food addiction. Back then, though, I couldn't see that the very things I was choosing to eat helped create and sustain my dependency.

Just like other addicts, overeaters display every symptom of addiction: obsession, compulsion, denial, increasing tolerance to their 'drug', withdrawal symptoms and cravings.

Unlike many other addicts, the compulsive overeater usually has this addiction triggered at a very young age, with the introduction of certain types of physiologically addictive, highly refined starchy/sugary 'foods'. This is therefore a deeply ingrained addictive pattern for many, with strong associations of comfort and security. Food and mood are intimately linked. Widespread obesity is just one result. Most people eat **far** in excess of their actual physical needs. As a society, we are *very* emotionally attached to food and overeaters take that to an extreme. The compulsive behaviour that characterises overeating is not logical and when these patterns intertwine with a diet of toxic, processed foods, obesity is an almost inevitable outcome.

Please remember that while the process of recognising addictions like this can be very helpful, the key purpose of such acknowledgment is to help us actually move *beyond* addictions and, most of all, the perception of oneself as a 'recovering addict'. This 'addict' identity can easily become a tag we identify with and become attached to, to the detriment of our fullest becoming. In making ongoing and increasingly positive choices, you are, in truth, an 'Active Transformer', freeing yourself and moving beyond the persona of 'addict'. Choose the perception of *Active Transformer* for yourself instead, and with it the delight of knowing that your life is consistently and progressively 'lightening up' with every positive choice you make.

So, Where Would YOU Like to Go?

Creating Your Optimal Vision...

Ideally, having read this far, you already have a clearer understanding of how you have been dealing with food. Plus, you're in the swing of including at least 50% raw foods into your daily intake by this point, right...? If not, you might like to re-visit the 'Are You Eating Raw Yet?' boxed section above.

With all that under our belts, it's now time to create your *optimal* personal vision of how you would LOVE to be interacting with food and life.

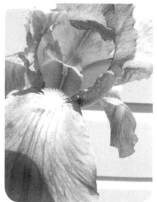

Mind Map

You might enjoy creating your Optimal Vision as a 'mind map' rather than by simply writing vertical lists on a page.

To create a mind map, you write down the subject of your focus in the centre of the page (e.g. 'my ideal emotional life') and draw a little circle around it. Then you jot down your thoughts and feelings on this subject all over the page, as they come to you. Later, you can add lines from the centre circle, radiating out like the rays of the sun, connecting to each of the ideas you've noted. You might also connect ideas that seem to relate to each other. This method often helps generate a clearer picture, as well as more creative responses than when we write in a vertical list.

Perhaps in the process of reading this far, you've found that you identify with a great deal of what has been put forth. You might feel heavy, sensing a lot of unhealed, complex history and patterning behind you. Yet that's where those patterns can remain, permanently, if you simply make a decision, decide to move outwards into a new way of life and take action. Leave behind any limiting thoughts like 'I can't do this/I'll never succeed/I'm always going to be overweight' and realise that you *can* make positive new choices.

You are the one who selects each thing that goes into your mouth and everything you choose to eat, in turn, builds your cells and influences your entire health and well-being. If you have decided that there are things you want to change, what are **you** going to start choosing intead? *Where do you want to go?*

A great way to kick-start this process is putting your vision in *writing*. That's what we're going to do in this section, using a series of simple guiding questions, which follow below. So, gather together a lovely fresh sheet of paper and some colourful pens.

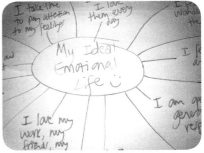

Understand that you can create health and joy for yourself at any level you choose. It is all a matter of choice and focus. We all have access to the same choices from the Universe. You want to eat only raw, organic, plant-based foods? Write it down. You want to weigh 130 pounds? Write it down. You want to inspire others to improve their health? Write it down. Open your mind and your heart and get clear about what **you** want to order from the menu of life. Choose abundance, health, joy, creativity, synchronicities, laughter, pleasure, acceptance. All these gifts and more are available to you in every moment, no matter what you may have thought before. Create your vision of where you want to go, then let go, with the faith that it will unfold in its own time (and not necessarily in exactly the way *you* might have expected...)

Sometimes, even though you may think you *know* many of the things you would like in your life, putting it all clearly into words or a vision feels a bit tricky. However, consciously taking time to write your vision out, remembering the truth that Everything Is Possible, is a very powerful thing and it's certainly something you *can* do. Your clear vision is a great friend for your progress. So don't skip this assignment!

The following questions and exercises are designed to help you clearly define your Optimal Vision for yourself. You don't *have* to answer every single question in each of the ten sections; they are there for guidance and to prompt your awareness. Remember that (other than the first section on 'How It Is Now') you are answering these questions from the point of view of your **Optimal** Vision for yourself, rather than how you feel and how things seem to be right now.

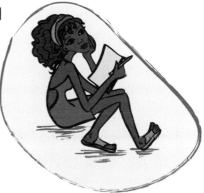

For this exercise, you might want to use a piece of beautiful paper, or a special notebook, as this Vision is something you will preferably keep and refer back to often. Be sure to write in the *present tense*, as if these things already exist and always use positive words and phrases such as 'I have/I am/I love' rather than 'I am not/I don't have/I cannot'. Using positive language and the present tense helps to affirm for yourself that these shifts are something 'real' – they are not distant dreams – they are things that hold real meaning for you and that you are now choosing for yourself.

HOW IT IS NOW:

How do you feel – physically, mentally, emotionally and spiritually – right now? Give three sentences to describe the way you feel about each of these aspects of your being.
*(For this section **only**, as you think about your answers, write them down in the past tense - e.g. 'I used to feel...')*

*Answer the rest of the questions below using the **present** tense, e.g. 'I have/I am/I love' and so on.*

YOUR OVERALL IDEAL VISION:

Imagine your 'ideal' life: how do you feel in this ideal life, physically, mentally, emotionally and spiritually? Give three sentences to describe the way you feel about each of these aspects of your being.

YOUR IDEAL PHYSICAL BODY:

Describe your ideal vision of your physical body. How does it look? How does it feel to be inside it? How does it move? Which new sensations can you identify? How does it feel to be healthy all the time? What do you feel when you see this body in a mirror? How do you keep this body active? How much rest and sleep do you get? What is your energy level like? How do you care for your skin? Do you feel attractive? What do you love about this new version of yourself? How much physical contact do you make with others? How often do you fast or cleanse this lovely body?

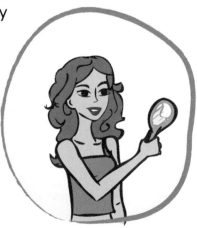

YOUR IDEAL MENTAL STATE:

Describe your ideal mental condition. How do you

see the world? What do you think about most of the time? How harmonious are your relationships with others? What social events do you engage in? Which activities do you LOVE doing? Which positive thoughts do you focus on daily? How is your self-esteem and confidence? How clear is your thinking? How well do you express yourself? How often do you laugh and smile? What inspiring media do you read/watch to support your positive thoughts?

YOUR IDEAL EMOTIONAL LIFE:
Describe the kind of emotional life that would be part of your ideal vision. How do you feel, most of the time? How often do you tell others that you love them? How do you handle challenging situations? How do you support others in their journey? How do others behave towards you? What brings you the most joy? How do you express your love to others and yourself? How does it feel to be balanced, happy and emotionally available? What do you feel passionate about? What does it feel like to be living your heart's desire? How do you encourage yourself to feel great consistently?

YOUR IDEAL SPIRITUAL CONNECTION:

Consider your ideal vision of your spiritual life: How is your relationship with your Greater Power/Spirit? Do you practice forgiveness, compassion and honesty? How often do you make conscious contact with your Greater Power/Spirit through prayer/meditation? How is your connection to your intuition – that 'still, small voice' inside you? How do you serve others? What kind of synchronicities flow into your life? How do you make use of the abundance you attract? How do you feel and express gratitude?

YOUR IDEAL RELATIONSHIP WITH FOOD:
What kind of foods and drinks do you consume in your ideal vision of yourself? What is your water supply like? Where does your food come from - do you grow it yourself? Which flavours and recipes do you enjoy? What is your kitchen like? How do you feel when you eat? What size portions do you eat? How many times a day do you eat? What time of day do you start and stop eating? How does it feel to eat with intention? What kind of blessings do you give to your food? How do you chew your food? Which foods help you feel fantastic?

YOUR IDEAL RELATIONSHIP WITH EXERCISE:
Which sports or activities do you love to do? How often do you exercise? Where do you exercise? How do you feel when you exercise? How does it feel

to be in a healthy, agile body? What activities can you do now that felt diffi-cult for you before? How often do you let your body heal with rest, massage and other treatments? How often do you stretch? How does deep breathing transform your life? How much exposure to the sun do you get?

YOUR IDEAL HOME LIFE:

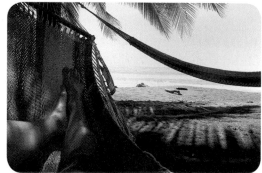

What is your home life like in your ideal vision? What kind of home do you enjoy? Where do you live? What is the air quality like there? Which facilities are nearby? What kind of social connections and community surround you? Who do you share support with? What are your intimate relationships like? How is your sex life? What do you do for fun? Which kind of music do you listen to? How is your home furnished? Where do you eat? How much support do you have for eating raw? Where do you go on holiday? What are gatherings in your home like?

YOUR IDEAL WORKING LIFE:

Which work brings you the greatest joy? Where is your bliss? What inspires you? How does it feel to do work that is fulfilling? How is your prosperity? Where do you work? Does work actually feel like play? How many hours a day do you work? When do you start and finish working? How much holiday and rest time do you enjoy? Which hidden talents are you developing? Which other people or charities do you support with your abundance?

IMPORTANT: If you find yourself 'fast-forwarding' to the next section without creating your vision, **press 'pause'**, get out the paper and do yourself a vital fa-vour - CREATE YOUR VISION! It's a *major* part of your positive becoming...

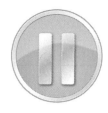

PLEASE do not skip over the above writing task and simply continue reading.

Once you have your Optimal Vision in place, take a few minutes to think about just what might be holding you back from already living this life, *right now*... Which limiting beliefs, fears, doubts and patterns currently keep you from living this Vision? Do you *truly* believe yet, for example, that you can do, be or have anything you desire? What would happen if you were su-per-healthy, happy, balanced and vibrant? What if there was no more illness, financial issues, gossiping, moaning and binge-eating? What then...? Could it be that there are some lingering, limiting beliefs and patterns that you might benefit from releasing...?

Our *true* beliefs strongly influence our outcomes in life. The Universe responds precisely to our beliefs. If these beliefs are not aligned with the life we are *stating* that we'd love to enjoy, we are unlikely to see the results we're looking for. For example, if you find yourself saying that you want to move to the countryside, yet your *true* inner belief is that this is never go-ing to happen, there is not yet an alignment between your Vision and your beliefs and the Universe will simply bring you whatever you truly believe. To bring your beliefs into alignment with your intentions, feed your Vision with positive, loving, joyful energy and thoughts. Have faith, keeping your 'eyes on the prize' of this Optimal Vision you have created for yourself, truly be-lieving that it is unfolding for you. It may very well be a case of 'acting as if', at first. Act *as* if you are someone who believes they **are** going to live out in the countryside sometime soon, if that is what you truly desire. Start to fuel that positive vision – focus on it, imagine what it's going to be like to live there, feel the joy you will experience in that space, as though you are there now, the things you'll see and do and so on. Refer back regularly to your notes from the exercise above, to keep yourself on track.

If, while reflecting on your 'Optimal Vision', you *do* identify any limiting beliefs within yourself that you suspect are holding you back in some way, it can help to note these in writing, though I encourage you not to *dwell* on them. (If you do write them down, I suggest using the past tense – e.g. 'I *used* to think/feel/believe'.) We are putting our attention consciously towards what we **do** want now, rather than what keeps us in patterns of limiting our potential.

> *"...you must decide if you want to act or react,*
> *deal your own cards or play with a stacked deck.*
> *And if you don't decide which way to play with life,*
> *it always plays with you."*
> *--Merle Shain*

Without creating your ideal Vision of where you want to go, you have nothing defined to head towards. You will be leaving your life open to ad hoc flow, instead of intentionally moving in a direction that is meaningful and joyful for YOU. I want you to get the most out of this process and to feel great, so I strongly suggest doing the above exercise. Even if it means you write down only one sentence for each of the ten areas of your Vision, that is enough for now – you can always enhance it later. Just get *something* down on paper, so that you know at least a little about where *you* want to go. This is *your* journey. Keep your Vision in a safe place where you can refer to it as often as you like and even add to it.

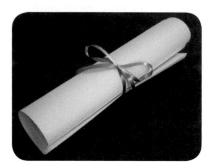

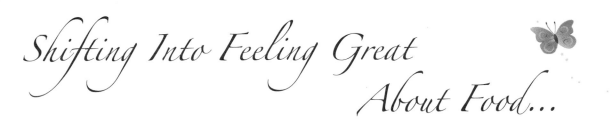

Shifting Into Feeling Great About Food...

Emotional Healing and the Raw Lifestyle

Eating raw can be considered one tool or pathway on a healing journey. In our modern societies, many of us live quite distant from direct contact with nature and this can impact our well-being in myriad ways. Going raw can then be a bridge from any disjointed, addictive patterns into active transformation on all levels, as we come more into alignment and reconnect with nature, simplicity and our 'true selves'.

If you are new to the raw lifestyle and curious to know more of the fundamentals about eating this way, please turn to Appendices A and B, where you'll find twenty top tips for eating healthily as a raw foodist, followed by ten simple, delicious raw recipes.

Beyond impacting the physical level, there are many ways in which eating raw can affect and help uplift our emotional, mental and spiritual well-being. This is what we'll be exploring in this section.

In the Long-Run

I want to make this absolutely clear from the outset: if you truly go 100% raw, in the long-run you will naturally come to require less food. There is no healthy way around this. As the body detoxes, it simply and inevitably becomes a more and more efficient 'processor'. Assimilation improves and you will therefore require less food to function optimally. Now, financially and in many other ways, requiring less food may, of course, sound great. However, *emotionally*, this can be very tricky for some people to handle. We come face to face with our compulsive food patterns and dependences. We may have changed the actual foods we eat, yet self-destructive *patterns* of eating persist. The body may require less fuel, yet we still compulsively want to eat large quantities. It becomes increasingly harder to ignore this contradiction the longer we stay raw.

While it is true that a raw lifestyle can be a fantastic tool for helping to shift one's focus from eating for emotional to primarily physical reasons, if you are not well prepared for those shifts, the impact can feel devastating. It is therefore highly advisable to have some solid alternative activities to turn to, diverting your attention from eating. We humans are virtually *always* looking for something to distract ourselves with. Before the going might even *begin* getting tough, give yourself a head start by experimenting with some of the 'spiritual' or emotionally-supportive exercises outlined in the Guidance section below. You will then have these already lined up as positive options whenever cravings arise, rather than turning to food. You will be creating a rich foundation for your transformation.

Off the Scale

Do you have a tendency to weigh yourself regularly and find that your mood is often influenced by the numbers on the bathroom scale? If so, I strongly suggest either giving the scales away, or at least cutting down your use of them to perhaps once a week/month. Obsessively weighing ourselves and fretting over each number seems far from beneficial for our serenity. Instead, pay more attention to the way that your *clothes* fit to get a sense of how your body might be changing. Weight constantly fluctuates, especially for women during each menstrual cycle. Keep in mind too that muscle weighs more than fat, so the number displayed on your scale may not really be telling you that much in terms of your health anyway.

Being raw can be an outstanding tool to release all that isn't our true self and 'shine up' all that IS our real essence. Almost everyone who goes raw encounters big shifts in life: jobs, partners, homes, etc., so there can be quite a lot of upheaval. This is not something to fear, however, but an absolute blessing to celebrate, as you move into a life that contains and supports the things that you actually love. The 'false' self falls away and your whole vibration and being change. It can take courage to pursue that, to follow your highest truth and stay with it: just remember you are not alone.

To ease the process, choose to focus first and foremost on *recovery* from self-destructive, limiting behaviour, allowing any desired weight loss to inevitably and 'effortlessly' unfold. Many overweight people focus on body image and seem to believe that losing the extra weight and being slimmer will be 'the answer to all their problems'. They might choose a mainstream diet to follow, for example, experience some weight loss, then find themselves shocked to discover that their 'real' issues that require healing are in fact still staring them in the face. Being thin has somehow not miraculously made everything OK. The fact is, *however* you lose the weight or keep it off, the spiritual malady still lies beneath the surface, awaiting essential healing. Without addressing the emotional and spiritual aspects of your transformation *as well* as the physical, you cannot expect to experience sustained and real freedom from the 'troubles' of your life. *Thinness* is not the hallmark of recovery or of a happy life. True happiness comes from inside us, not from wearing a certain dress size. We don't have to wait until we are a target weight or size before allowing ourselves to experience good things.

If someone does try to ignore/bypass the emotional and other aspects of their transformation that arise, they usually end up feeling 'stuck' in some way. This may manifest as yo-yoing endlessly back and forth between cooked and raw foods, wanting to be 100% raw and thinking you can't maintain it, or simply feeling depressed. This discomfort arises when our behaviour jars against our highest truth. When we ignore the messages from within and don't explore things for release, it's easy to feel out of alignment and stagnant. By starting out on this path of transformation, it's like you've given your body and whole being permission to begin releasing old 'waste'. This includes emotional waste and now it is time to process it. This can be a *prime* opportunity to readjust aspects of your life – if you choose to see it that way.

Sometimes people feel they 'just can't handle' exploring their transformation on all levels, yet the truth is that we can get through *anything* if we choose to, especially with support. The more people who choose to step into integrity and transform, the more support there is for everyone to release the old paradigm of a society that seems to be based around fear and distraction.

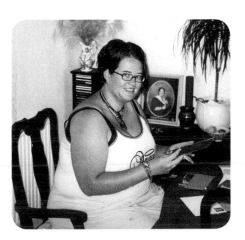

I completely understand that, at times, it may *feel* very challenging to be on this kind of raw healing journey; yet overall, I believe wholeheartedly, through my own experience, that the benefits can truly outweigh any perceived disadvantages. If you commit to enjoying your healing, get support and work through any issues as they arise, you *will* witness a wonderful transformation. Let's face it, at the start of *my* raw journey, I was nearly 300 pounds and had no interest in health or well-being whatsoever. Yet as I write this, I have stayed on this path of active transformation for over six years now. Would I still be doing this if the rewards were not fantastic? It's just a matter of choice...and I truly believe that...

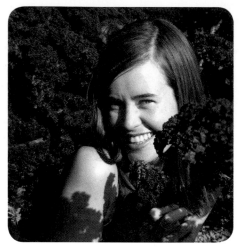

If I can do it, anyone can!

Is Food Your Entertainer?

On reflection, most modern humans seem to have quite a peculiar relationship with food, which could benefit from some re-evaluation. It usually comes down to this:

We treat food like entertainment.

We pick up food if we're partying, lonely, celebrating, miserable, upset, rewarding ourselves, anxious, seeking comfort and so on. Yet these situations have little to do with the primary purpose of eating food: fuelling the physical body. We've become so detached from nature and our true sense of self that we no longer clearly perceive the real role of food in our lives. Instead, we've made it our 'entertainer/comforter'.

As an example, let's take someone who is feeling very lonely and withdrawn. Eight o'clock in the evening comes around and their loneliness expands into a huge sense of emptiness. Rather than looking *inside themselves* at their patterns and starting to take action to create a different life path, they make a beeline for the kitchen and emerge with a big bowl of popcorn. We so often reach out and grab food, trying to make it fill a gap it *cannot* fill. Doesn't this seem like an odd and illogical scenario, from the outside looking in? If someone with this kind of relationship to food then goes raw and carries these behaviour patterns with them, things can get really messy. Going raw is, in many ways, like pressing the 'release' button in your body and life. As you stop taking things into the body that clog it up, your cells finally get the chance to 'exhale' all the waste that has been building up for years.

The body always moves towards optimal health and efficiency. Over time, it will come to ask for simpler and 'cleaner' combinations of foods, as well as less food. If you ignore these requests and instead keep using food for entertainment or comfort, you can run into many

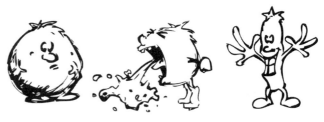

A clogged cell 'exhales'

health issues, including bloating, gas, drowsiness, lethargy, pimples and more, as the body struggles to handle all the excess and unnecessary food.

When we view life mostly as a series of opportunities to eat, we miss out on so much of the real richness that we can experience here. Without a deep and rewarding relationship to the Universe and community around us, many of us reach out to food as a substitute, even though food is neither intended for that purpose nor close to a match for so much else that is on offer in life. It's like using a band-aid on a gaping wound that really needs stitches. As a quick cover-up, it might seem to help in the short term, yet it leaves the deeper wound still waiting to heal. If we don't address and resolve the core situation (in this case, our dependence on food as a substitute for a deeper connection to life), our unhealed issues can easily multiply.

As we have seen, we arrived at having such a strong *emphasis* on food in our societies through myriad ways. For a start, pretty much everyone eats, so food is an easy commodity to sell. Advertising for processed foods is highly visible throughout our media and in public spaces. Food is legal, often cheap and widely available. Parents use it as a quick way to quieten/reward their children. People share food socially. The list goes on. It's easy to see how we can develop such an affinity with using food, sometimes to the degree that it is almost a reflex action.

However, let's be clear: food does not = fun. It's a fuel that keeps you vibrant and alive to HAVE fun. You can also of course *have fun* when you eat; it can be fun, for example, to try exciting and tasty new raw recipes or enjoy occasions where food is available as part of the festivities. Naturally it's also wonderful to see people delight in their new raw explorations, rather than moaning that they 'can't eat bread anymore' and so on. Essentially, the point is to choose to NOT make food the *centre of your world*, your primary source of fun and the thing you turn to for comfort. There are so many other more effective and enjoyable ways to address and express our emotions than by eating, as suggested throughout the 'Guidance' section. Slowly, slowly, we can move into a space where we *really* know how to entertain and enjoy ourselves, beyond food.

> **Let's make food something we simply consume,
> rather than something that consumes our lives.**

This kind of clingy relationship with eating as our source of fun is not to be confused with the 'preoccupation' with food some of us experience when we first go raw. Usually, at the start of being raw, there can be quite an intense learning curve, with lots of new information to assimilate. It's common to feel like your attention is often on food-related matters. However, as this re-education process starts to settle down over time, the focus on food can feel less directed, if we are willing and ready to release this. So this temporary preoccupation with food can be seen as a different thing entirely to *constantly* feeling fixated on foods as our source of 'fun'.

Finding the Balance

As we've learned, food addictions and imbalances do not simply disappear when one goes raw. It's common for people to carry unhealed compulsive patterns over into their raw lifestyle. There are certainly things about being raw that can help to release patterns that no longer serve you. There are no guarantees, however, that being raw = an end to food issues.

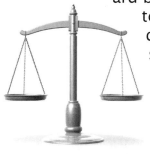

We've learned that when we stop eating highly processed foods like standard bread, pasta, cake and so on, the *physiological* addiction to those toxins is broken. Those foods have been helping distort and suppress our real feelings for years; now it seems we can free ourselves from such food-based emotional discord. The raw foods we eat instead can also genuinely nourish us, help clear up our blood stream, balance our blood sugar levels, clear up our brain fog and free us from sudden and sometimes disastrous mood swings. So in some ways, it seems it's easier to feel more balanced and happy and to eat less. That's great in theory and for some people going raw, it works impeccably. Often, however, coming off those heavy addictive processed foods like bread, we can hit major emotional detox. Binges can easily follow as an escape route.

We're used to spacing out and numbing ourselves with things like refined sugars and the sedating opioids in bread, pizza, cakes and so on. Without that kind of continued intake to 'medicate' our feelings, stuff down the stress and keep us hazy, we are faced – perhaps for the first time in our lives – with confronting our real feelings. So, instead of reaching out for our favourite cookies or candy to numb out when we start to feel uncomfortable, we now have new choices to make.

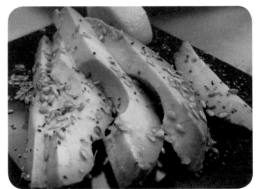

Again, some of us will turn to complicated raw recipes or heavy, high-fat foods like nuts, seeds and avocados to (unconsciously) try to weigh ourselves down and avoid connecting with our emotions. We may also typically eat large amounts of these foods or many heavy meals in the space of a day. These foods take a lot of energy to digest, so can divert focus away from our emotions, yet they really don't numb us in quite the same way as the processed, toxic foods. We are still left with more 'raw' emotions to deal with than might feel comfortable.

Your body is releasing old, stuffed-down emotions, just as surely as your cells are throwing out old physical waste. On top of that, you're also learning new things about how to handle your *current* emotions (if only from reading this book). This ongoing process can feel like a challenge. Get support from others who understand what you are experiencing; speak honestly about what is happening for you; breathe deep and use any of the other tools shared below to help you work through things. Remember that you are not alone and you *can* get through anything that comes up for you.

Many people do choose to turn away at this point, however. The prospect of facing their true feelings and no longer medicating themselves with processed food feels too overwhelming and they slip away from the raw lifestyle. This is surprisingly common even among those dealing with life-threatening illnesses who learn about going raw for healing. They may *say* that they don't want to die and will 'try anything' and yet, when it comes down to it, they actually don't want to live without the foods they're addicted to, so they choose to turn away from this healing path.

Another factor that can stump some people arises when they start to 'un-numb' themselves, only to feel 'confronted' by a society that seems so deadened emotionally that it feels painful to even **be** awake emotionally and tuned in. This is another reason why many simply put their heads back in the sand. The truth, however, is that if you do start to un-numb yourself and diligently hold and nurture a loving space towards those you encounter, you will start to see shifts around you and that loving space you have been holding will be reflected back to you many times over.

So, how do we find the balance between eating raw and coping emotionally? Thankfully, the longer we're raw and omit the most toxic foods COMPLETELY, the easier it gets. Our food issues become much less about avoiding our old toxic 'Trigger' foods and more about seeking and enjoying balanced patterns *within* our consumption of raw foods. If you *do* still find yourself bingeing on raw foods, it can at least be *less* harmful overall than bingeing on processed/cooked foods, although bingeing of any kind is not a recommended strategy.

For many, a classic stumbling block with going raw is the notion that 'if you're raw, you can eat everything you want, still lose weight and feel great.' While this certainly holds true to a degree (especially in the very beginning), statements like this tend to ring alarm bells for me... If someone uses that kind of reasoning, for example, to binge-eat three pounds of dates in one day, then that really doesn't seem healthy or balanced to me. Transferring **compulsive behaviour** from one way of eating to another is not the aim here.

 If you binge, this indicates that you are acting compulsively and suggests that you are in avoidance. Is there something that is not being expressed or addressed? Ask yourself this and turn to the *Raw Emotions* 'Guidance' section for help in addressing whatever comes up for you.

What we are ultimately aiming for overall is Moderation. If we can create a gentle consistency in our new lifestyle, this is a great gift to ourselves in terms of balance and serenity. For many, this is easier said than done - being consistent and balanced with *anything* in life can seem challenging. Aim for regular, gradual improvement rather than obsessing. Find a balance of slowly incorporating the new into the old that feels comfortable to *you*. There are many tips in the 'Guidance' section to help you create a stable new framework – use them! Also remember: it is what we do **most** of the time that really counts, rather than any little blips here and there.

Raw = Healthy, Right?

Eating raw is **so** radically different from the 'junk' that most people usually eat that it's easy to understand why people think it must be fine to eat anything as long as it's raw. Over time and with experience, though, it becomes clear that the picture for optimal health is much more refined than this. Just because something is raw, doesn't mean it's the greatest choice for our health, especially in large quantities. You can still be left feeling drained, puffy and spacey after eating raw meals. You can even (re-)gain unwanted weight. Raw food is still *food*, even if it's not what most people are used to fuelling themselves with. Just as with other foods, at some point the 'calories in/calories out' equation comes into play. If you are under the illusion that raw food is some kind of magical elixir that you can eat endlessly and indiscriminately, with no complications, you might find some issues popping up for you.

It is possible to technically be eating 100% raw and still not be eating in a very healthful way. For example, you could be eating many packaged or

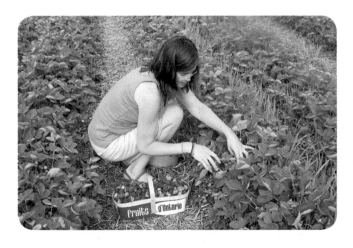

gourmet raw foods, like crackers, dried fruit treats, cakes, raw chocolate and raw pizza all day long. There is unlikely to be much fresh, living content in this kind of menu, so someone eating like this is unlikely to feel great in the long-run.

Try to imagine, in contrast, a paradigm beyond all packaged foods, where everyone eats simply from the Earth, gathering their food directly and eating it immediately. In that kind of situation, someone who eats raw cakes, crackers and pizzas all day long would seem a little odd, yes? It is only because we're so *accustomed* to eating complex and packaged foods that eating lots of 'gourmet' raw foods may seem comfortable for us, at least in the beginning. As ever, just because we *can* do something, doesn't necessarily mean it's the greatest choice for our health.

Raw Food: the 'Healer'...?

Another common misconception that often goes hand-in-hand with 'you can eat whatever you want, as long as it's raw' is the idea that 'raw food heals us'. It is not the *raw food* itself that heals us, or even the fact that raw food has more enzymes. It is the fact that we *finally* stop putting so many things into our bodies that are damaging, clogging us up with toxins and other debris. Your *body* does the healing by itself, once you stop adding in so many obstructions.

I no longer get ill. This is not primarily 'because' I eat raw food; it is because I don't put so many things into my body that are obstructive and cause disease. There is a big difference.

Similarly, a squirrel or other wild animal is not healthy *because* he eats raw food; he just doesn't consume things or quantities that are toxic and cause disease. Being well is our *natural* state; disease is not.

As mentioned above, I could 'technically' be eating raw food all day long and still feel terrible if I'm eating masses of 'raw junk food', oils and nuts, to the exclusion of, for example, fresh and vibrant green vegetables.

It can take time, though, to reach a place where we feel balanced with our raw food intake. There is no pressure to do it 'perfectly', right from the start. More dense/gourmet raw foods can be great stepping-stones towards a more vibrant, lighter lifestyle. Just have the awareness that, as a raw foodist, over time you will come to require simpler combinations and less food, to feel optimal.

Take, as an example, a 28-year-old who has been eating a 'Standard American Diet' their whole life. They will have 'levelled out' with this way of eating. They've had a lot of practice at it and most likely eat roughly the same kinds and quantities of food each day. If they then go raw, it's like a whole new ball game and they may feel as though they no longer know what to eat, how much to eat, or when. It will take time to 'balance out' with this new way of life too. It may well be close to five years or so before they feel really clear about what works well for them, on a daily basis.

What are the some of the rewards of doing all this? Well, as our bodies become 'cleaner', more alkaline and free from the dizzying influences of processed foods, pesticide residues, factory-farmed meats and so on, we often emerge feeling lighter, more calm and peaceful. Perhaps we have more interest in others around us; we're more open, loving, accepting and active. We can see more clearly what we'd love to be directing our energy towards and we take steps forward. We question things, experiment and enjoy; we are not passive participants in life – we are explorers.

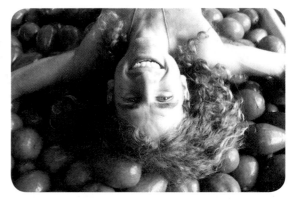

Few of us really make much use of the power of thought; most peoples' thinking tends to be clouded and numbed by low-grade food (refined grains, processed sugar, etc.), pharmaceuticals, 'negative' patterns and societal conditioning (including the strong influence of television). As we eat more raw food and less 'toxic' food, our brain fog starts to shift and lift and we start to see and question more the nature of our reality.

On the way, as we have discussed, a wealth of emotions often unfold to be healed – the main theme of this book. Along with all the information you are accessing here, your other great ally can most certainly be a community of like-minded individuals...

Raw Food Community

I strongly recommend reaching out for great support on this journey from other like-minded 'explorers'. Do not underestimate the value of support. The reason why groups like Alcoholics Anonymous are so prolific and successful at helping people is the support they offer from others who are on a *similar path*. Most people in our current societies are immersed in processed/cooked food addiction. It can seem very daunting if you feel like the only one swimming 'upstream' while everyone else is gushing on down past you. Help yourself out by connecting with others who seem to be on the same path as you.

You might even find it useful to ask someone to be a mentor for you on your transformative journey. Identify someone who inspires you and 'has what you want' in terms of the lifestyle, health, vibrancy and joy that they seem to

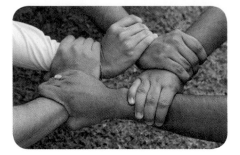

embody. Ask them to share their perspective with you so that you can learn from their experiences. Speak to them regularly and be open to what they communicate. It is said that we are 'the sum of the five people we spend the most time with', so who are *you* sharing your time and energy with...?

Occasionally, people embarking on this transformative journey can experience a lot of bitterness rising up inside them. They may think, 'Why wasn't I brought up like this in the first place? Why do I now have to learn this whole new way of living, by myself? Why was I lied to? Why was I sent to mainstream school?' and so on. Using the many tips in this book can help you work through and release any such resentment. Realise that holding on to bitterness serves no-one. Work through what comes up for you and move on, keeping your 'eyes on the prize' of how you really want your life to be – your Optimal Vision.

There is no need to ever 'go it alone' with your raw journey. I believe one of the reasons many raw foodists do not currently tend to live much longer than their cooked/processed peers is social stress. Modern raw foodists can easily feel isolated, awkward or strung-out, especially if trying to handle detox alone, in a speedy city environment.

Although interest in raw foods is expanding at an unprecedented rate, as yet there is little infrastructure or mainstream understanding for this simple way of life. Consequently, some people experience being raw as a struggle and yo-yo back and forth with it. Linking up with fellow raw enthusiasts, to share and support, is invaluable.

I hope the time will come when books like *Raw Emotions* will be obsolete museum artefacts because humans will have shifted so far forward into alignment with more natural ways of being. People will giggle at the notion that such things were ever perceived as needing to be explained in a book. Communities everywhere will be eating simply, from their gardens, enjoying their life paths and feeling balanced... This can all become manifest, if you choose it. Keep it clear in your head that, whatever anyone else may tell you, by taking this healing path you're actually 'going sane' rather than 'crazy'. There *are* other people out there who understand; connect with them.

If you are reading this book from within a 'citified' environment, where you don't feel very connected to nature, I'd like to share here a part of my own Optimal Vision. This is something I see as a *vital* component in moving towards greatly improved personal and world health.

To The Land...Spade in Hand

We are blessed to have a strong, positive shift currently occurring in the collective consciousness. People worldwide seem to be waking up more and more to the value of 'greener' lifestyles, including organic farming, alternative medicine, raw food, recycling, permaculture principles, renewable energy sources and more. Being 'green'/environmentally friendly definitely seems to be gaining popularity. As a result, even though it may not always seem so, it's becoming easier than ever to connect with others who are on a healing path.

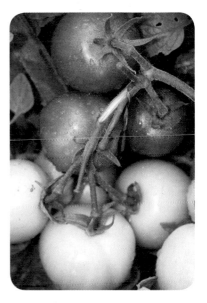

I see the brightest vision for our collective future at present as one in which as many people as possible get to the land and start growing their own food, using organic/biodynamic/permaculture principles. The benefits of this are far-reaching, from protecting our food sources, to being and feeling more directly connected to life, to regenerating the soil and the whole ecosystem. Act now and get your goodies growing, from heirloom and organic seed sources. Even if you only start growing a few things (lettuces, cucumbers, tomatoes) and plant them in pots/windowsill boxes, these are steps in a very positive direction, which you can keep expanding upon later. Be sure to also give your plants lots of love and attention - they are highly sensitive to human thoughts and actions.

The 'Anastasia' series of books, mentioned earlier, contains hugely inspiring information and imagery about growing our own food. Anastasia gives precise guidelines on how to grow foods and design a garden that will optimally serve each person. Most modern people are distantly separated from their food supply, growing little to nothing themselves. This is another feature of the kind of society we've been living in, where 'natural' things can seem remote and disjointed. Gathering food from your own surroundings has become the exception rather than the norm. Instead, people work long hours daily in jobs they often dislike, to receive some pieces of paper (money), which they then take to a brightly lit store full of packaged/lifeless food, that has often been shipped thousands of miles. They hand over some of the paper in return for these 'foods', most of which clog up their bodies with toxins. Who is benefiting here? Compare that scenario to people who are living on a piece of land where they grow their own produce. They simply pick food and eat. Which lifestyle seems to make more sense to you? The more people who get active and start growing food, the more support there will be for this grounded, loving and 'natural' way of life.

Many of the current practical challenges involved with 'being raw' directly reflect the way we've created societies that encourage people to disconnect from the land, consume poor-quality food and stay hooked in the same system. Imagine how much easier life could potentially be as a raw foodist if you and all those around you were growing your own produce and living more or less self-sufficiently from the land. Doesn't that sound like it could be a more joyful and fulfilling way of life than the standard nine-to-five office, commuting, getting-money-to-take-to-the-supermarket-and-pay-the-mortgage routine...? Hmmmm, I think so...

If you've had enough of being numbed and dumbed with poor-quality foods, it's time to take spade in hand and dig for victory...

Let's take a look at the following analogy. In the wild, a tiger is naturally 100% raw and is likely to be very healthy. Imagine taking the same tiger and keeping it in an artificial environment such as a zoo, while still feeding it 100% raw. It's going to be a lot tougher to keep the tiger calm than if you feed it a combination of raw and cooked/processed foods. The cooked/

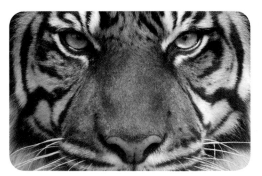

processed items can help to 'numb' the animal to its environment and keep it docile/more obedient/manageable. The same is true with domestic pets: people 'dumb them down' with kibble and so on, so that they're more manageable in the artificial home environments we inhabit. Now, while it's unlikely that most people feed their pets with that kind of objective clearly in mind, whether these actions are *conscious* or not, they can still be regarded as part of the same system.

The very same scenario applies to contemporary humans. We frequently numb ourselves with processed/cooked foods, we lack vital energy; we routinely stay 'in the system' doing things we don't truly enjoy, responding to advertising and media, living in artificial environments and so on. Through our choices, we have helped to contain ourselves in a particular system. By the same token, we can also make *new* choices and shift ourselves out of this system and beyond, to a life where we feel more genuinely connected and joyful.

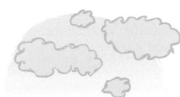

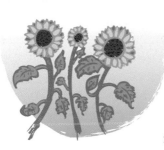

Going raw sets you off on a journey towards more simplicity and truth, nurturing a real connection with nature again. You might find that you want to go and live outside – for example, in the woods or by the sea. You may find that being in cities and the 'civilised' world starts to feel increasingly uncomfortable to you. Eating more food straight from the Earth can help return us to a sense of our true essence.

There are degrees of involvement in such shifts, of course. The more wild, freshly foraged foods you eat, for example, the more likely you're going to want to reconnect to the land. However, you certainly *can* live on shop-bought raw foods in busy cities, eating at raw restaurants and so on; it's all a matter of choice.

Many folks who maintain a raw lifestyle in a stressful city environment soon sense that they feel unsatisfied and uncomfortable there; they feel moved to make further changes. With a cleansing raw lifestyle, the body detoxes and wants to keep moving *onwards* to the next level of more vibrant health. If you resist this impulse by continuing to live in a toxic, stressful environment, eating mostly pre-packaged, dense raw foods, you may find that you experience weight gain, develop degenerative diseases and so on, just like many others who live in such places.

This is one of the key reasons why some people stop eating raw, although they may not realise this *consciously*. The lifestyle calls them forward, to step into a place of more authentic connection with themselves and the Earth and they are perhaps neither ready nor willing to make that move. It may feel as though there is 'too much' to let go of, dissolving so much of the familiar structure they have been part of, plus they may not want to experience such upheaval.

Feeling this discomfort, they may assume 'eating this way just doesn't work for me' and revert to eating less raw. They *choose* to stay in the toxic environment, rather than move onwards into the more vibrant health they *could* embrace on their raw path, in less toxic surroundings. Yet would a zebra, for example, ever metaphorically seem to say, 'Raw food doesn't work for me, I'll just whip up some pasta instead'...? The environments we choose to stay in can have a substantial influence on our food choices and health in general. Choose where you live with care and take note of ways in which it seems to affect how you feel and the choices you make.

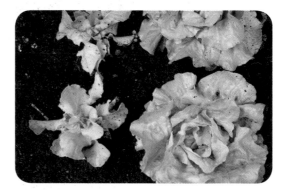

The raw path is shining brightly right now to help people move towards simplicity and reconnection with the Earth. It's one aspect of a significant revolution in consciousness, in which we can all actively participate. The more people who engage in this lifestyle, the more overall demand there tends to be for organics, raw foods, eco-friendly products in general and so on. When increasing numbers of people start to *want* to grow things themselves and spend more time in nature, the wonderful knock-on effects are blissfully abundant... So, whether it's a flowerpot, a window box, a garden plot or more...touch the Earth, befriend the land, take spade in hand and get to it, Active Transformer!

Conscious Connections

Our lives are filled with choices we make; in our current times, what we choose to *buy* and *use* are potent reflections of our preferred lifestyle. We can all bring our consciousness into our every consumer choice, from organic cotton clothing to solar power, vehicles that run on 'green' energy, eco-friendly paints, furnishings and more. You vote with your dollar with every purchase you make; thus buying 'green' can help you to feel good about your contribution to the economy and world health. Eco-friendly products may seem a bit more expensive at first, yet just think about the overall higher value of them from the larger perspective. As you shift your habits away from purchasing cheaper, often poorly made, pollution-contributing products towards a greener lifestyle, your sense of healthy connectedness to all life will surely accelerate. If the idea of 'buying green' is a new concept for you, I highly recommend watching the wonderful twenty-minute video entitled 'The Story of Stuff', to help facilitate this shift in your own life. (See http://www.StoryOfStuff.com.)

A happy resurgence in community living also seems to be currently under-way, with countless vibrant ecovillages forming worldwide. (Again, a great number of these communities are inspired by the ideas shared in the 'Anastasia' books.) Many people feel understandably isolated living alone in city apartments, or raising children without extended family. Choosing to live instead in a community with other like-minded people, sharing ideas, child-care, celebrations, seeds for growing food and so on, can be an enor-mously enriching shift. These communities need not be strictly organised, by any means; perhaps a collection of family plots, closely located, which allows people to connect with each other as they like. Each family/individual has their own piece of land and housing, plus there may also be shared com-munity spaces for gatherings. Indeed, it is often considered ideal for *each individual* over the age of around thirteen to have their own dwelling/space, so that there is always somewhere private for each person to go in times of reflection/integration or to release tension. When people come together into communities in this way, the potential seems much greater for feeling more connected to nature, at peace, understood and supported. (For more information about growing your own food and living in communities, see the Resources section below.)

So, there you have a glimpse of part of *my* 'Optimal Vision'...

Isn't it *Boring, Eating Raw?*

This is one of the questions I get asked most often about raw foods. People

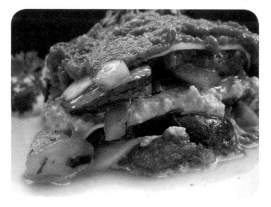

going raw commonly fear that they will no longer have much variety of food choices and it will be 'boring'. The truth is that you can make raw food as gourmet and taste-bud-tantalising as you choose; it's all about your choices, perspective and outlook. Being raw, like everything in life, can feel as exciting or 'dull' as you like. If you **choose** to see what you're doing as positive and abundant, you'll likely enjoy it much more.

Accustomed as we are to having thousands of different packet foods available, our taste buds are used to massive over-stimulation. In contrast, going raw may at first just seem bland. Yet the idea that these packaged, processed foods are actually *different* to each other is, in many ways, an illusion of advertising and marketing. Most of them contain the same kinds of ingredients – wheat, sugar, dairy, artificial flavourings, etc. – mixed and packaged in different ways. If this kind of 'variety' is really the equivalent of choosing between different additives, preservatives and chemicals, is that truly what you want for yourself?

It often seems as though we're addicted to combining many different foods and flavours as we eat. A meal of scallops, followed by grilled steak served with a pumpkin bisque and sautéed potatoes, rounded off with a chocolate torte and whipped cream might sound like a chic, classy meal to many humans. Most *wild* animals, in contrast, seldom eat more than **one** thing at a time and the *variety* of foods they ingest is pretty small. Cows eat mostly grass, for example, sharks eat different fish, squirrels eat lots of nuts and so on. Humans, on the other hand, have contrived whole industries out of combining different foods and revelling in the 'variety'; yet how conducive are these combinations really to optimal health?

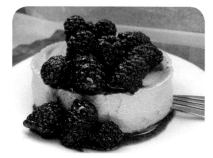

I'm not suggesting that we all switch over to mono-meals (eating only one kind of food at a time – e.g. a meal of just mangoes) and be done with it. Particularly in the beginning of going raw, eating 'gourmet' foods like raw pizza, raw chocolate pies and so on can be a huge comfort and defray any initial feelings of deprivation/boredom. However, usually, the longer one eats predominantly or totally raw, the body effortlessly and steadily moves towards feeling *just* as satisfied (if not more so) with simple food choices and our interest in the more complicated meals falls away...

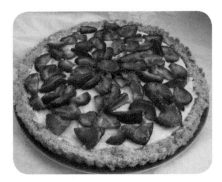

"Nature never produced a sandwich."
--Dr. Tilden

So, eating raw may *seem* 'lacking in variety' and 'boring' when we first start

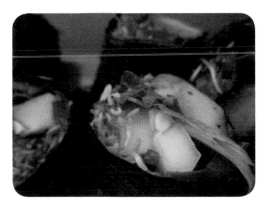

out, yet the more we delve into it, the more we might see that, in fact, this is just a matter of perspective... There is no need whatsoever to fear that it's all tedious carrot sticks and drudgery from here on. You can create the most incredible gourmet recipes with raw foods, if you want. There are countless raw recipe books out there for inspiration – see the Resources section for more info. (Please note that all the pictures in this section are raw food creations from the ext-RAW-dinary Terilynn at thedailyrawcafe.com – check her site out for tasty raw recipes.)

Once we peel back the illusion that eating cooked/processed foods means more excitement and variety, we can step into a whole new awareness of how raw, natural foods can truly satisfy us.

Personally, my whole outlook flipped when I went raw. The items in boxes and cans, which were once the only things I was really interested in, no longer even look like food to me. Instead, the salads and greens I used to mock as 'ridiculous' are now my much-loved staples – it's all just a matter of perspective.

I love to guide people towards viewing their raw lifestyle with a positive outlook. This is an amazing gift we're giving ourselves. It can all be about abundance and joy, if you choose for it to be. I often hear people who are raw saying in miserable tones something along the lines of 'I can't eat that because I'm raw' or even more astonishingly, 'I'm **not allowed** to eat that because I'm raw'. ***Not allowed***...? Who took that permission away??? There is no law that says, for example:

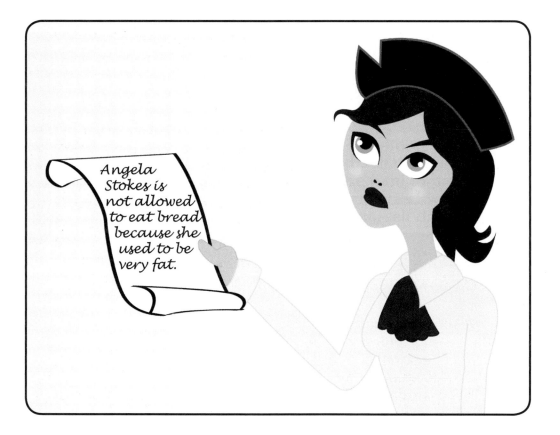

Angela Stokes is not allowed to eat bread because she used to be very fat.

I just don't choose to eat things like that because they look toxic to me. It is my **choice** and I love it. How you *feel* is extremely significant. Do you feel good about your raw lifestyle? Are you enjoying it? Or are you moaning about what you 'can't' eat? It is all a choice. Embrace and celebrate *your* incredible lifestyle choices.

What Am I Really Hungry For?

Learning to tell the difference in your own body between 'true' hunger and 'emotional' hunger is a very useful skill. Most people in our societies eat *far* in excess of their actual physical requirements. When we get the impulse to eat something, we can so often assume it's the stomach talking rather than the mind. If you look closely at what prompts you to eat, it can indeed be tough to figure out where the urge is coming from. Do you really 'need' this food that you desire, to be physically nourished and well? Or is it just your mind asking for something to distract itself with, for emotional satisfaction? This conundrum tends to be especially difficult to fathom when we first start out raw.

Here's a tip for how to tell whether hunger is coming from the stomach or the mind: reflect on *what* it is you want to eat. When we are truly hungry, we usually feel like we could eat *anything* (of course, usually within any pre-defined dietary boundary, such as 'any raw vegan food' for a raw vegan, for example). If, on the other hand, your 'hunger' is directed specifically at 'that' piece of raw carrot cake (for example) and you're not really interested in anything else, this tends to suggest that the hunger is coming more from the mind. The mind *wants* to have the experience of eating that cake, even if your physical body isn't really ready for it.

> *What the mind wants*
> *isn't necessarily beneficial for the body.*

The physical body works always towards optimal health. The mind, however, seems more interested in habits, patterns and experiences and may insist that you 'need' a doughnut, for instance.

Another way to establish if any hunger you feel is 'true': wait half an hour and see if the physical sensation in the stomach intensifies, if indeed there even *is* a feeling in the stomach (which is a big clue in itself). If, after half an hour or so, the feeling of hunger has grown, then you're almost certainly experiencing 'true' hunger and it's prime time to eat. If we eat when we are *not* truly ready for it, we're asking the body to do extra digestive work, along with adding more material to the body that is simply not needed.

Now, this all sounds very logical; however, we may run into issues when we try to actually incorporate these concepts into our lives. Many of us simply *do not like* feeling hungry – in fact, we've made a point of avoiding it as much as possible. The truth, though, is that feeling hunger is a natural signal from the body, letting us know when we're ready to bring in more nutrients and fuel. It's nothing to fear and thankfully, the longer we are raw, the more we tend to adjust to these natural body rhythms; it also gets easier and easier to understand the messages from our body. It may take many years, yet over time, we get progressively more adept at recognising 'emotional/mind hunger' for what it is and refrain from acting out on it and eating.

These 'false hunger' sensations are not to be confused with intuitive desires from your body for certain foods at certain times. For example, you might find that one day all you want to eat are red berries – they just taste and smell and look so good to you. This is your body's natural wisdom working to heal itself; it's very likely there is something in those berries that your body could really use right now, like antioxidants or iron. If you check in with yourself during a day like this, you'll likely find that you are actually *physically* hungry at the points when you want to eat – it's not just a 'mind game' driving you to eat pounds of berries. These kind of intuitive longings for certain foods tend to naturally become more clearly defined and easier to interpret, the longer you are raw. It is simply not as easy for the body to 'speak the language' of toxic, chemical-laden products with you, mainly because these 'foods' contain confusing ingredients, rather than simple nutrient compounds that the body can recognise. If your intake consists of Twinkies, sodas and hamburgers, for example and you've never eaten a goji berry in your life, how is your body going to know to ask for gojis for extra B and C vitamins when it wants them?

In my first couple of years as a raw foodist, I reacted to any feelings of hunger with the same response: I ate. I wasn't tuned in to my body enough at that point to sense where signals came from. These days, my understanding is much more refined and now I can clearly recognise the difference.

When I experience the desire to eat something, I check in with myself about it. I ask myself a few quick questions to determine if the hunger is truly physical, such as 'when did I last eat?', 'has that food digested yet?', 'how much water have I had so far today?', 'would I eat some other raw vegan food right now other than what I'm thinking of eating?', 'how long have I *had this sensation – could I leave it to see if it intensifies?' and so on. I also ask myself if I would feel good eating something very simple right then – like watermelon. If my body doesn't seem to be ready to eat **that**, then I'm certainly not going to ingest anything more complex.*

Based on the answers to these self-enquiries, I decide whether to eat then or not. Usually, in the space of any given day, there will be times when I experience 'emotional hunger'. Nowadays I just acknowledge it, smile and move on with my day. It is a relief for me to not get caught up in the 'drama' of emotional eating and you don't have to experience it either...

A 'Quick-Fix' Cravings Guide

In the section below called 'Healing the Emotional Connection with Food' (pgs. 120-133), you'll find details of the powerful three-step approach I recommend for managing and releasing cravings and 'false' hunger. In addition, here is a list of twenty quick 'trouble-shooting' tips, in no particular order, for handling cravings or desires to overeat, as they arise:

* H.A.L.T. - This is a slogan from '12 Step' groups, such as Overeaters Anonymous. It stands for 'Hungry, Angry, Lonely, Tired'. If you feel cravings/ bingeing coming on, HALT and ask yourself, 'Am I hungry, angry, lonely or tired?' If you're hungry and it's a while yet until you'd planned to eat again, drink some water, breathe deeply and also consider that perhaps your food intake could use some adjustment. If you are angry, lonely or tired, recognise that *eating* is not a practical solution for any of those feelings. For example, if our body really needs some *sleep* to **re–fuel** our batteries and instead we eat, we just create more digestion/assimilation work for an already tired system. So, before reaching out impulsively for food, remember to 'HALT' and consult the Guidance section of this book too, for more supportive solutions.

* **The Bigger Picture** - If you feel like you're on the brink of a binge, you might find it useful to ask yourself how you think you might feel after three hours, if you DO act on the craving now. Taking a moment to see the bigger picture like this, instead of just diving in, can sometimes help us put things into perspective. We might feel more able to release the urge for *instant* gratification in preference to feeling good in the long-run. After all, in the long run, does it really seem 'worth' eating (processed) foods that we're addicted to if the result is dysfunctional health, especially in later years?

* Drink Water - Often, what we've learned to interpret as hunger is, in fact, thirst. Most people are chronically dehydrated. Whenever you feel hunger or cravings, make it a habit to drink at least a full glass of pure water. You may find that the hunger/craving vanishes... Other 'phantom' hungers can

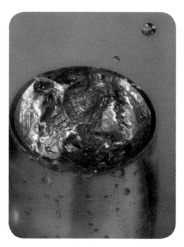

result from eating lots of fatty/salty foods *or* foods that have not digested well; we might get odd sensations in our physical body that we interpret as hunger. Again, if we wait for a while or drink some water, we'll commonly find that these sensations dissipate.

* Drink Tea - Drinking warm teas can be very useful for pacifying emotional hunger/cravings. Reaching for a cup of warm, caffeine-free, herbal tea as an alternative to any 'Trigger' foods, can help you to feel that sense of warmth, comfort and satisfaction, without the burden of a food binge. This is especially useful if you are in a cold climate, plus it's extra hydration for the body and can bring the bonus of some great nutrients. I recommend teas such as ginger to warm, rooibus or peppermint to soothe, pau d'arco for anti-candida properties and so on. Some raw foodists don't drink warm teas, for the same reason they don't eat warmed foods. I like warm tea though and feel it's a useful tool for certain times; perhaps just don't use *boiling* hot water.

* Negotiation - If you're dealing with strong craving/binge patterns and it seems clear that you are going to eat *something*, a useful strategy can be 'negotiation' with yourself about *what* you consume. Check in with yourself to see if you're open to alternatives. If, for example, your mind seems to be screaming that it wants cake, you might enquire as to whether it's really just the *frosting* on the cake that is grabbing your attention and would bring satisfaction. If so, eating only the frosting rather than the whole cake could be a form of 'damage limitation' if it's obvious that you're going to eat something regardless. You may even be able to negotiate with yourself from 'cake' all the way to 'a banana' or something similar instead, if it becomes clear that all your body really desires is some kind of sugar/fuel. Perhaps you could even get from 'cake' to 'a hug' instead – then you really see healing in action.

Only **you** can know in each situation what is truly going to work for you as a real point of release for the craving. Each incident can be a complex mix of physiological and psychological yearnings and you are the only one who can sense for yourself what will feel satisfying. Replacing cake with a banana, for example, because you think it's the 'right' thing to do, then finding that you eat the cake anyway twenty minutes later is not necessarily very beneficial overall. Of course, ideally it's preferable to not end up in 'negotiation' with ourselves at all on these matters. This kind of negotiation is certainly not suggested here as regular practice; it is intended more for 'emergency' situations where it becomes clear that you are going to eat *something* and there's a chance you could make it easier on yourself.

* Sniff vs. Snack: Aromatherapy - It can be very beneficial to 'feed the senses' on another level when we're in a phase of strong food cravings. Instead of repeatedly interacting with the world through our sense of *taste*, we can focus instead, for example, on our sense of smell and nurture ourselves with delicious aromatherapy scents. You might sniff essential oils, burn incense or scented oils, or take a luxurious, pungent bath. Our senses of smell and taste are intimately linked, so if you find a scent that really pleases you, it might help you simultaneously sidestep the desire for edible satisfaction. The scent of vanilla is said to be very good for helping people handle food cravings. (You could also seek out relief through the other senses: touch, sight, hearing. Check the Guidance section for more ideas along those lines.)

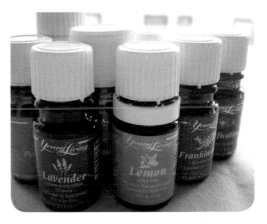

* Colon Hydrotherapy - This is a practical process that some find very useful for handling cravings. Colon hydrotherapy helps release the flow of old waste that's being dumped into your system as you cleanse. As mentioned elsewhere, going raw is like pressing the 'release' button in your body; the old toxins/food particles get thrown out into the bloodstream and colon. Colon hydrotherapy can help us to swiftly move those things out of our bodies, so that we don't keep 're-toxing' ourselves with them, remaining stuck in addictive patterns. Colon cleansing is also simply a healthy practice for the whole body. If you can distract yourself away from thoughts of bingeing and instead actually end up *releasing* more waste (rather than adding more in), this can help you feel a whole lot better about your choices. You might choose to receive professional colonics from a licensed practitioner, or do your own enemas at home. Either option will help relieve the pressure and release old waste. We sell a range of enema bags in the RawReform Store.

* Get Perspective - When you're gripped by the intense desire to keep eating after a meal, you might feel compelled to act out on such strong feelings, *right then*. However, if you allow yourself a broader perspective, you'll likely see that you actually go through this same pattern at almost *every* single meal. There is nothing 'unique' about this individual moment of intensity, this is just the pattern you've set up and keep repeating. One way to get more perspective on what is really happening in **intense moments** is by taking a pen right then and writing notes about what we're experiencing, or speaking our thoughts into a recording device. Then, the next time we feel that intensity, we have something to refer to – a point of reference to help us see the truth of this pattern and realise that we don't *have* to act out on it. We can acknowledge what is happening and respond to the 'demands' of our mind kindly yet firmly, as we might with a child, e.g. "Thank you, dear mind, for the suggestion to eat more. The body does not actually require more fuel now, we'll eat more again later." If you keep choosing to *not* overeat like this, the feelings of compulsion will start to fade.

Women often also find it beneficial to track cravings in line with their *menstrual cycle* or hormonal fluctuations. Keeping even brief notes about days and times of day when cravings seem intense can help you to build up a picture of your patterns over time and see if you notice any correlations with your body cycles. For example, you might come to realise that your strongest cravings *always* come when you're pre-menstrual. When you have greater perspective on these patterns, it can help you to feel more at ease in the moments they arise. If you find yourself suddenly intensely fixated on bingeing, for example, you can stop and reflect on how this fits into any pattern you've noted so far, rather than feeling each time like it comes 'out of the blue'.

* Reach Out - If you're on the brink of a binge, try reaching your hand towards the phone, rather than the fridge door. Speaking with *someone else* about what is happening for us can make all the difference, helping us to step outside the circles in our heads. A phone may not even be necessary; maybe at the end of a meal with a loved one, you feel compelled to keep eating. Expressing your feelings about this may help you to end the meal then, rather than 'acting out' and eating more than you'd intended.

* Ask Questions - At the end of the section above on false hunger, I wrote a little list of the questions I ask myself if I feel hungry and focused on eating. You can ask *yourself* those kinds of Qs too if you're feeling a sense of urgency about eating something. You can inquire gently: when did I last eat? Has that food digested yet? How much water have I had

so far today? Would I eat something else right now, other than what I'm thinking of eating? Remember that cravings come *and go*; this too shall pass. Instead of jumping in with a knee-jerk response to a craving, we can step back and ask ourselves a few quick questions like this, to gain a clearer perspective on what's happening.

* **After-Meal Activities** - Having activities planned for immediately after meal times can be a great incentive for ending a meal. This doesn't necessarily need to involve *physical* activity, just something to help draw you away from thoughts of eating more – perhaps a phone call to a friend, tidying up a drawer or writing a letter. Planning activities that are far away from the kitchen/location of food in your home is a good idea.

* **Plan of Eating** - One of the most reliable tools for dealing with cravings and false hunger issues is to follow a daily Plan of Eating, as outlined on pages 124-128. If you make and follow a structured Plan each day of what you're going to eat, it can be a powerful aid in averting sudden emotional binge sessions.

As you adjust to your new way of eating, be sure you are also getting *enough* nutrition, or cravings can easily follow. For optimal health, consume neither too *few* nutrients nor too *many*. Finding *your* place of **moderation** and consistently following the 'middle path' is the most advisable. Be open to adjusting your intake as you move along your path of transformation, finding out what works for you.

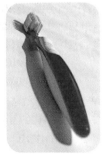

* **Brush Your Teeth** - Here's a simple, handy tip for those who find it hard to stop eating after a meal: brush your teeth and you're less likely to want to keep eating, with a mouth full of minty-fresh whites...

* **Give Thanks** - You can reinforce good feelings around your food choices by thinking to yourself with gratitude at the end of a meal something such as, 'Wow, what a feast that was', rather than the common 'Well...that's it, I guess...' that many food addicts dread. This can help in situations when you've finished what you intended to eat and your mind seems to be asking for more. You could even get a plate or bowl etched with a beautiful message such as 'I feel nourished, satisfied and grateful for this meal', so that as you gradually clear your plate, this message is revealed, helping you reaffirm your intention to honour your eating Plan.

* **No Picking** - I highly recommend not 'picking' at parts of a meal while you are *preparing* it, as this can easily lead to eating much more than you'd planned. Instead of nibbling at things as you prepare food, opt for beginning to eat only when you're relaxed and settled with a complete meal ready in front of you. Also, if you have any leftovers, be sure to store them away somewhere, rather than leaving them out where they are visible; remember the saying 'out of sight, out of mind'!

* **Take a Break** - If it feels like your eating patterns are off-track and far from where you'd love them to be, you might find it beneficial to take at least 24 hours out from your usual routine, for a Juice Feast or fast. Taking a short 'breather' like this, to break up the cycle of eating can be a huge relief. We can re-gather focus and reset our intentions, before easing our way back into eating again. *Please note*: while taking a day or so out to fast/Feast like this can be useful on an occasional basis, overall we are aiming for balance and *consistency* within our daily eating habits. The intention is not to end up bouncing backwards and forwards between fasting mode and bingeing. Please use the option of fasting/Feasting responsibly, with great care and attention.

* **Fingers and Teeth** - Keeping our fingers and/or teeth 'busy' with something other than eating can help us to not binge. You might employ your fingers, for example, in some knitting, puzzle-work or plant-tending. Chewing on raw licorice sticks or sugar cane stalks might keep your teeth entertained. You can also purchase 'jaw exercisers' that help keep your mouth engaged, while simultaneously strengthening your jaw and teeth. If our fingers and teeth are already involved in activity, we might find we're less likely to reach out for food.

* **Timing** - If it feels useful to you, consider working with a time schedule for your meals, to keep on track. (This is not recommended for everyone: for some people, this can feel too restrictive and lead to rebellion. If you sense rebellion in yourself, leave schedules aside – this is just *one* tool among many!) You might like to plan starting times for your meals, or possibly *finishing* times, if that helps you to wrap up eating and step away from the table. If you do use a schedule to structure your eating, I recommend not getting *overly* rigid and attached to it, as this can create extra tension. Leave space for some flexibility, while doing your best to honour your intentions.

* **No 'Overlapping'** - Setting the intention to not 'overlap' our meals, in terms of digestion, can help us to side-step cravings and overeating. The concept of 'not overlapping' is explained in more

detail in Appendix A; it basically means only eating when you're sure you've finished digesting any previous meals, so as not to overlap digestive processes. This tip may not necessarily make so much sense to you at first. In my experience, people tend to relate to this idea more over time, as we tune more into the messages from our bodies. At some point you might notice, for example, that you honestly want to eat only when you feel 'true' physical hunger. True hunger cannot be present if you're still digesting food in the stomach. This might help us to handle cravings as they arise, along with the desire to *overeat* at the end of a meal. We might feel less inclined to keep on eating *now*, if we realise that by doing so, we're unlikely to get genuinely hungry again today (or even the next morning, if we're eating late at night). Put simply: the sooner you stop eating a meal, the sooner you'll get hungry again!

* **Journalling** - Use the power of the written word to help keep you on track. If you're feeling low about your eating habits, get pen to paper and write down exactly what you're feeling and thinking, right then. Similarly, at points when you're feeling very clear and focused about your eating (often first thing in the morning), make notes – what are you feeling at this point? What are you thinking? What are you eating these days? What are you *not* eating? How much water do you drink? These written notes can be invaluable if you find yourself in a sticky place with your food choices again. In challenging moments, you can refer to these notes for a bigger perspective on your patterns and hopefully find the inspiration to stay on track.

Another useful exercise to try when you are in a clear, steady space, is to do some writing about overeating. How does overeating seem when you are in this balanced state? Making such notes might help you to start feeling more like an 'observer' of the often impulsive and irrational action of overeating. It can even seem *absurd* to contemplate overeating when we are in that space of stillness and calmness. The more we can separate ourselves from that impulsiveness, the less likely we are to act out, when we next feel the pull to overeat.

You may also find it useful to use **visual cues** in your journal, such as old photos of yourself, a picture that captures your optimal vision for your life, grocery receipts or anything else that helps inspire you to stay on track.

In addition to these tools, the Guidance section (pgs. 162-216) is packed with useful suggestions for diverting your attention away from any intense desires to eat, eat, eat...

Is Being Raw Necessary for Sound Emotional/Spiritual Health?

Clearly, it is entirely possible to lead an emotionally balanced, 'spiritual', connected life without being a raw foodist. Millions of people worldwide live in this way. Being raw is by no means a necessity. Our food intake is just one piece of the puzzle, not *the key* to feeling connected – though it can be a significant aid to enhancing all aspects of our lives, including our emotional and spiritual well-being. For a healthy, happy life, it seems more vital to have *love* in your heart than raw food in your belly. It's not all just about eating food that hasn't been heated over 118 degrees...

That being said, eating raw food *can* certainly bring us more into alignment with nature and simplicity. A deeper sense of connection almost inevitably follows. While I thoroughly believe that it is *possible* to think so positively that one can literally live on junk food and be healthy, since the *feelings/energy* that we impart to food are so vital, I also believe in and have experienced a simpler approach. If we consume junk food while in a space of total love, gratitude and enjoyment, for example, we can transmogrify the structure of that food and still be nourished. However, very few people alive at this point seem easily capable of doing this and it uses a lot of energy in the long-run. It seems altogether simpler to eat food that *naturally* aligns us with a healthy body and connection to the planet: high-vibrational, raw/living food, straight from the Earth. Eating food that is already simple, fresh and unadulterated, means there is no need to transmogrify denser foods.

The energies carried in the foods we eat are also *quite* significant, especially as those foods then become part of us. Taking food into your body that has been grown, harvested and prepared with *love*, preferably by you or someone healthy you know, easily ensures a nourishing vibration from your intake. Feeling connected to your food is very enriching.

If you eat mainly organic foods, you can usually assume they've been grown with more love and consciousness than conventional produce, which may be handled by any number of people who are far from living their passion in life. Personally, I am happy to pay more for foods that have clearly been

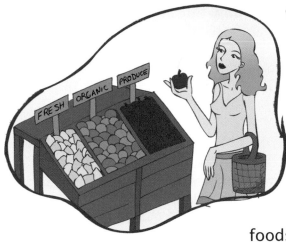

grown and handled with loving attention, rather than getting a larger quantity of cheaper, 'empty-feeling' produce. Life is all about choices and we vote with our 'dollar' every single time we purchase things. I want to feel great about the choices I make, the businesses I support and the foods I eat, so that's why I buy organic whenever possible.

We can also add to the high vibration of foods by giving blessings and expressing gratitude before, during and after eating.

In short, it is by no means *essential* to eat raw foods to enjoy a sound emotional and spiritual life. However, eating raw, organic, loved-up foods is another tool that can make it so much easier to feel connected.

Love Changes Everything...

I want to share a little story about how the power of love can have a huge influence on the foods we ingest.

One friend of mine has been very high raw for decades, with periods as a 100% raw foodist. Even now, when he visits his mother, he will eat a little of whichever cooked foods she offers him. This is not due to any kind of cravings – it does not excite him to eat those things. It is, for him, an act of love.

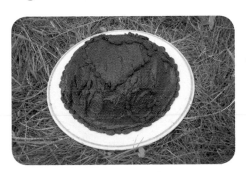

He knows the love that has gone into making that food. It is held out to him with excitement and joy, by someone who loves him dearly. The energy in that exchange can be enough to **transcend** any or all potential ill effects he may otherwise feel from consuming, for example, baked goods. In this case, he is more interested in the loving energy of the situation than a cold, hard nutritional analysis of what is being consumed. This is a clear illustration of how our feelings are vital in terms of our health, happiness and even digestion. When my friend eats his mum's cake, it is not from a place of 'ignorance' or indifference about nutrition. He is fully conscious of the general impact of processed/cooked foods. He is simply choosing to enjoy the flow of love instead: he feels good, she feels good, everyone's happy.

Also, since he eats very high raw the majority of the time and has done so for decades, occasions like this are mere 'blips' in his journey. He eats a little cooked cake, then he's straight back to simple raw foods. His body can handle it – it is what we do MOST of the time that counts, not the little blips. Now, if he were eating very high raw then 'sneaking off' to the local baker once a week to get his fix on doughnuts or something, that would be another story. Do you see how the energy of that scenario is very different? If he's *feeling* shame/guilt/worry about the cooked foods that he eats and thinks that he 'needs his fix' of doughnuts, the effect on his well-being would be very different. It would be coming from a place of fear and addiction in him, rather than love. It would feel toxic. Do you see how someone can, on the surface, be performing exactly the same action – e.g. eating a piece of cake – while the *experience* they are having is vastly different? Depending on where the motivation comes from, the consciousness regarding this and most importantly, how you *feel*, the experiences can be poles apart.

I hope that this anecdote is not taken as 'license' to nonchalantly eat processed/cooked foods whenever you desire: it simply helps illustrate the point that often there are interesting dynamics at play, over and above the nutritional content of food. I still believe that for *most* people, *completely* omitting items like refined sugars and processed starches is optimal for health.

*Personally, I would not choose to eat anything at this point that is not raw. I do appreciate my friend's approach to this matter though and believe that the **energy of love** has the power to transmogrify anything. I simply don't feel good about processed/cooked foods at this point in my life, even if they do seem to be offered with love, so eating them would not serve me well right now. We all have different paths and choices. In my life nowadays, most people around me are raw, so I actually seldom encounter these kinds of social situations anyway - and for that I am grateful. However, if you are wondering about the dynamics of socialising with people who aren't into eating raw, the next section might interest you...*

Being a Raw Foodie in a 'Cooked' World

One of the main issues that raw people report is feeling uncomfortable if they decline food offered by others. I fully understand this feeling. It can seem awkward and even disruptive to refuse food at social gatherings, especially if it's offered with love. There are many ways you might choose to handle this.

One approach is to accept small amounts of whatever's offered, as in the anecdote just discussed above. Perhaps you eat the food, perhaps not. Often, simply the act of accepting into your personal space a piece of what is offered is enough to appease the situation, without drawing attention to yourself or creating tension. You can always leave it on a plate or give it back to the Earth for composting.

Some people choose avoidance tactics when offered processed/cooked foods, such as saying, 'I already ate' or 'I don't feel well at the moment, thanks anyway' and so on. These are simple ways to diffuse the energy of the situation. How-

Connecting with the Raw Tribe

None of my blood family are raw, but they support what I do and have made some adjustments to their lifestyles since seeing the changes in me. For that I am grateful.

I feel so blessed to have a WONDERFUL raw partner, who lights up my life with incredible support, care and love. He is a beautiful, gentle, generous man and has been raw even longer than me. He makes yummy raw food, takes me on magical surprise trips and always speaks his truth with me. I am so grateful for the love we share. Aside from him, I enjoy connecting with a vast network of beautiful (mostly raw) friends, all over this globe.

Wherever we go, people welcome us into their homes and communities to share our stories. To me, this feels like the 'tribe' we belong to - our fellow soul group - and I love connecting with all these incredible beings as we travel. It's delightful to share space with others who are enjoying the same kind of lifestyle (rather than asking questions like 'Where do you get your protein...?') Most people I interact with these days are raw. I have met literally thousands of raw foodists now and feel extremely blessed to be able to travel from one raw home to another on this journey.

Even if you don't know any other raw foodists locally and you're not much into travelling, there are plenty of ways you can still reach out and connect with others on this path. See the Guidance and Resources sections for more details...

ever, you might not feel comfortable with such tactics and want to express your truth...bravo! A word of warning, though – this can easily whirlwind into myriad discussions/questions/confrontations and so on. If you prefer not to engage in repetitive explanations of your food choices, you might elect to give a simple, gracious 'no, thanks'.

Some raw foodies feel that if others don't accept their way of eating, their relationship is perhaps not genuinely based in unconditional love, support and acceptance. They may decide to cut off contact with such people. This can be a great strain socially and is not a path I would really recommend. There is room for acceptance, love and understanding on *all* our behalves. If, for example, you attend a barbeque gathering where most people are happily *enjoying* the food and proceedings and you spend the whole event writhing inside with bitterness and judgement about their choices, do you really feel you're contributing much love to the occasion? Or to your own health? You are no more able to make their food choices for them than they are for you. Do your best to let go, breathe deeply and radiate love to all those in your presence, regardless of whether they're eating grilled steak...

If you are used to **preparing** food for others, who are not interested in coming along the raw path with you, this may also feel awkward. I recommend

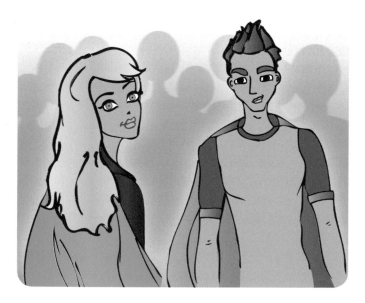

making the food you feel good about for everyone - for example, a BIG salad - then letting others add in whatever else they want, alongside that. This seems like a great compromise; you are providing things you feel good about to those you love and they are eating things that please them.

A great way to expand your social life and feel like less of an 'outsider', is to socialise with other raw foodies. There are quite a lot of them around, once you start to look... You'll find suggestions and links to support groups who organise raw gatherings in the Guidance and Resources sections below. Get ready to replace those burgers and beers with raw chocolate and durian!

> *"Time spent attempting to change others affords little time for personal change."*
> *--Georgette Vickstrom*

One key point I love to share about social issues is to **Be The Change**. Something I see happen repeatedly when people go raw is that they get very excited about this lifestyle and want to tell everyone around them and *change* everyone else too. The truth is, we cannot change anyone else or make their choices for them. People need to come to this and choose it for *themselves*, in order for it to really get integrated in a way that's meaningful for them.

When someone is being a 'raw evangelist' and trying to convert everyone around them, it will often backfire and send people in the opposite direction, which I find very sad to see. Force only yields *temporary* compliance, then quite the opposite effect can occur and people recoil. This is a common pattern with children and spouses of those who go raw.

I feel the best thing we can do to share this healing message is to simply **be the change**. Inspire others with your *own* genuine delight in this lifestyle. Live your life as a happy, vibrant, healthy raw foodist and people will start to come to *you* and ask for guidance. They will see your glow and want to know where it comes from. This, to me, seems to be the optimal time to share and the greatest use for your energy flow. Let the questions of those who are *interested* guide your sharing, rather than trying to control and force interest in people who are resistant.

I understand that it can feel painful to see those we love consuming foods and doing things that, to us, seem very detrimental. However, rather than trying to manipulate them into doing what *you* want, try **letting go**, breathing deeply and picturing in your mind your greatest vision for their health and happiness. Remember, love changes everything...

Healing the Emotional Connection with Food

So, how do we get back into a space where we feel good about our relationship with food again? How do we create that rhythm where we feel as good as we can, as often as we can? How do we move from the 'Realisation', through the 'Transition', to the happy state of 'Maintenance'? How do we start to unravel that crazy tangle of habits and patterns inside of us? There are a number of steps we can take, which will be discussed in the following sections. You'll read about my three-step approach to breaking addictive patterns with food, along with a great number of tools and tips for working through the emotional issues surrounding food.

It is, after all, our mental/emotional relationship with food, not the food itself that can make it seem tough to eat optimally. If it were simply the food itself that was the 'issue', we would see all people reacting to all foods in exactly the same way. That is not the case.

Our habitual eating patterns, peer pressure, unconscious needs, cultural patterns and so on drive a huge part of our consumption. When we can distinguish between these and our healthy intuition about what, when, where and how much to eat, we are on a great pathway to healing.

Once we have identified any non-functional food patterns that detract from our well-being, next comes the choice to let go of them... Herein lies the big question. Are you ready to let go of the patterns that no longer serve you? You can discover ways to do that, right here...

How to Break Your Addictive Patterns with Food

In my first (e-)book, *How to Go Raw for Weight Loss: An Introduction for Overeaters*, I introduced three simple tasks for those dealing with addictive patterns around food. These tasks are adapted from suggestions offered in the Overeaters Anonymous fellowship. I'm repeating *my* version of these exercises here (with a few minor updates), as they've been extremely powerful for helping thousands of people relinquish the foods and habits that do not serve them.

(N.B. You might like to use a new, clean notebook for these writing tasks. Honouring your new lifestyle in this way can feel very nurturing and provides a clear place to keep your notes together.)

Task 1: Examine Your Past

Dedicate some time – just fifteen minutes or so at first, if that's all you feel you can manage – to taking an honest and searching look at your personal history and patterns with food. First we illuminate the destructive aspects of our eating habits, then we can eliminate them, once we know what we're dealing with. This is such a simple task, yet it's something few people seem to actually try, without prompting. Our eating patterns seem so entrenched that we simply 'take them for granted' and don't examine them.

Here are some questions you can begin asking yourself, to guide your writing:

When did I start overeating?
What were the circumstances around me at that time?
How did I feel during and after overeating?
What was it that I overate?
What do I overeat now?
When do I overeat now?
Which foods do I crave...?

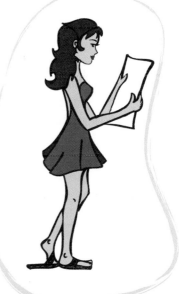

If you do not identify yourself as an *overeater*, feel free to adapt the questions here so that they feel more suitable for your particular history.

Here are some suggestions:

Are there any foods I suddenly started eating a lot of, at any time?
What was happening then?
Do I find myself suddenly eating that food again in similar circumstances – for example, if I'm upset?

Was there a time when I started to use food in a way that now feels un-healthy to me?
What were the circumstances around me at that time?
How did I feel when I ate in that way?
What was I eating?
What are the main things I eat now?
When do I eat now?
Which foods do I crave?

Writing down the answers to these kinds of questions (so you can refer back to them again) and even sharing your findings with others, helps to clarify any eating habit issues. You can use this process to help you realise the ways in which your relationship with food so far may not have been very healthy. For example, taking some moments to note what was happening at a time when you pitched into odd eating habits can help identify 'Trigger issues' that could use some healing. Far from simply using food as fuel for the physical body, many of us are heavily involved with food emotionally. We can use the information gathered through this exercise to move forward and create new patterns for ourselves.

Task 2: Trigger and Vigour Lists

Write a list of your personal 'Trigger' foods – the foods you have a strong preference for, which set off cravings and compulsive eating patterns. These are the foods you'll need to omit to arrive at real recovery – and every person's list is different.

Your list may include:

*things you eat in large quantities
*things you start eating and just can't seem to stop
*things you eat to the exclusion of other foods
*things you eat in secret after hoarding and hiding them from others, or turn to in celebration, sorrow or boredom.

'Triggers' tend to be refined foods that are sugary, starchy or fatty, high in calories and low in nutritional value. This list can be as specific as you choose, e.g. every different type of chocolate bar you crave, or you could simply list 'chocolate' – whatever feels right to **you**, in order to be completely clear about your own Triggers. (For most people reading this, the Trigger List will consist largely of processed/cooked items. However, if there are *raw* foods you also identify already as Trigger items for yourself – for example, dates, honey or almond butter – please do list those too.)

Write out your Trigger List *right* now – don't procrastinate on this important step. It only takes a few minutes and then you'll have a good overview of your eating habits. Being very honest when writing your Trigger List allows you to see exactly which foods to let go of/surrender for optimal health. You will also very likely be able to see clearly the *key ingredients* that recur throughout the items in your list. Most people notice, for example, that refined white sugar and white wheat flour are common ingredients in their Trigger List foods. This is a clear indication that foods containing these ingredients are best left out of your intake from now on. Your Trigger List will be a valuable tool over the weeks and months to come. Refer back to it whenever necessary to remind yourself which foods 'trigger' you, especially if you feel your boundaries are blurring.

The good news is that, along with your 'Trigger List' of foods that you're better off omitting, you'll also have your very own 'Vigour List' of things that are great for you to include. So, along with your Trigger List, be sure to also make your Vigour List of the *raw foods* you already enjoy that help you feel vibrant. Maybe you know that you love plums, spinach and pumpkin seeds, for example; if so, write them on your list. These are the things to begin adding more and more of to your intake as you continue on your raw path. Be sure to try to get as many green leafy veggies that you know you like onto your Vigour List especially, as these are major healing foods for us: balancing, energising, alkalising, re-mineralising. You may also find it useful to add in any non-raw whole foods that you enjoy for your Transition, such as steamed quinoa, brown rice, cooked hummus and so on.

Your Vigour List foods will help you to 'exercise' your taste buds and retrain them into enjoying natural tastes. People who are used to eating toxic processed foods often find it hard to even sense the taste of raw foods at first, as their taste buds are so used to being blasted with all kinds of intense chemicals and flavours. Your Vigour List will help you move into a healthier lifestyle confidently and enjoyably and it will almost certainly grow as you explore and discover more and more raw foods that you love. From the outset, have it *at least* in the background of your consciousness that your Trig-

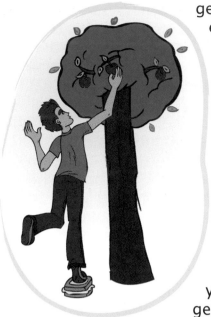

ger List contains the items you are heading towards eliminating *completely* from your intake (preferably sooner rather than later). If you don't feel ready to eat high raw right now, I recommend that you simply start adding in *more* items from your 'Vigour List' (which you know you love), preferably eating at least 50% of your intake as fresh raw food, from the outset. It is important that the new way of life you are embracing feels comfortable to *you* and 'meets you where you are at'. Focusing on 'restrictions', things you 'can't eat' and what you are going to 'give up' is not conducive to feeling empowered. However, if you keep adding in more of the vibrant, fresh raw foods you DO like, you'll usually find that your body asks for more of the same and the Triggers naturally start to lose appeal...

The Vigour List is the antidote to your Trigger List. It is your new 'prescription' and ally in moving towards a more vital, vibrant life filled with vigour. It can be really useful to post up your Trigger and Vigour Lists somewhere visible, such as side by side on a sheet of paper stuck on your fridge door. This way you have them easily available to re-read as and when that serves you. You can keep your food choices inspiring, healthy and delicious by referring to your lists often and also adding to them. This way, you'll be more likely to stay in the game.

Use your lists as well to help shape a shopping list that you feel good about. Then when you do go out to buy food, aim to stick to the list you've made and avoid shopping on an empty stomach.

Task 3: Making Your Plan of Eating

Once you have your eating history/patterns written out and your Trigger/Vigour Lists, you can begin to make a daily 'Plan of Eating' for yourself, one day at a time. A Plan of Eating is your 'personal guide to nourishing foods in appropriate portions'. You can use your Plan to create *structure* and to approach food in a calm, balanced and rational way. Drawing on what you've learned about your patterns so far, you know which behaviours, foods and key ingredients to exclude completely from your Plan, for optimal well–being. You also have your Vigour List to help guide you to create meals using (raw) ingredients you love. Then, on a day-to-day basis, you can make a simple personal Plan of what, when and how much to eat. You follow that Plan, one meal at a time, one day at a time.

With your eating Plan, you eat exactly what you've intended for the day – nothing more and nothing less. This allows you to stop relying on shaky statements like 'I'll just have one of these...' and develop instead a solid, reliable Plan, in advance. Your focus will start to shift towards eating to fulfil your physical needs, rather than emotions.

With a Plan, you'll almost certainly find that the amount of time you spend thinking about food decreases dramatically. You write your Plan down, share it with another if possible, then forget about it until it's time to eat. **Free from obsessing** about food, you can devote a much clearer head to other enjoyments. For a food addict, eating can easily become the top priority in life, with everything else feeling like an inconvenience. Directing so much energy, time and thought towards food can feel truly crazy-making. Any overeater who has, for example, stood in a party pretending to listen to someone while eyeing the buffet table, silently waiting to slip away for yet another feed, will understand the relief of dropping these patterns. Thus, a Plan of Eating does not equal a *loss* of freedom; rather it leads you to freedom (though your *mind* may try to tell you something different). With a Plan of Eating, you can release old behaviour that doesn't serve you and try a new approach. Understand that everybody's Food Plan is unique and will also likely change over time. That is natural; we are all on our own journey. Simply find what serves you best and enjoy it.

What better time than now? Begin today! Write down exactly what you intend to eat today, share the Plan with another person (if possible) and then consume only those things that you've written down, one meal at a time. You may or may not find it useful to note the times of your meals. You may also find it rewarding to take a quick review of your Plan at the end of the day and affirm for yourself that you followed through with it. At the same time, you can take a quick mental review of whether you felt *genuinely* hungry before eating, plus how you felt emotionally before and after each meal. Paying attention to details like this can help us understand more about how our healing is unfolding. Keep reading for tips later in this chapter on how your Plan of Eating might look...

Plan of Action

I recommend making your Food Plan in the morning, before you start consuming *anything*, other than water. In the morning, we're fresh to the day and most people find they tend to make 'cleaner' food choices this way. Many can identify with making 'hazy' food choices late in the day, so, making a Plan of Eating at that time is best avoided. It's also much easier to know, on waking, how you feel that day and to tune into which foods you'd like to enjoy, rather than trying to do so the day before.

Refrain from dramatic thoughts of doing this 'forever' – this is just about *today*. Just for today, eat only those things you listed for yourself. If, by the end of the day, you find that you've remained true to your Plan of Eating, then congratulations – you've just had your first day free from compulsive eating. Then make a Plan again tomorrow…and the next day…and the next…

There's a saying that 'not having a plan is like planning to fail'. While I choose not to see anything in terms of 'failure', I know for myself that trying to navigate the food terrain of a day without an adequate Plan feels unnecessarily draining to me. It's just SO much easier to make a Plan beforehand. Compare it to going on a road trip to a place you don't know and doing *nothing* before to prepare – no map, no 'MapQuest' directions, nothing. Consider how much more time, energy and resources you would be likely to expend trying to find your destination that way, compared to taking a few minutes before the trip to jot down some directions. Making a Plan of Eating is exactly the same principle. It takes just a few minutes in the morning to outline your food choices for the day and that's it, you're done and your brain space and energy are freed up for other pleasures. It's simple and, most importantly, it *works*. Countless thousands of people worldwide find that this little idea makes all the difference for their health and happiness, where no other 'diet plan' has ever helped them.

There are usually people who want to know how long they '*have to do this for*' before they can stop using a Plan of Eating. You do not have to do anything – the Plan of Eating is just a suggestion. However, if you are using it and it's working for you, I would recommend that you simply keep on using it, one day at a time.

The thought of a *lifetime* of no more corn chips may seem too awful to bear right now. Similarly, you're unlikely to feel inspired by telling yourself grimly that you're now 'on a Plan of Eating *for the rest of my life*'. We can take these pressures off by thinking only about <u>today</u> – 'just for today' – we can do something for 24 hours that may seem impossible to imagine doing for a lifetime. The past is gone and the future is not yet here – the only thing we have is the present moment, today – and today we can choose to use a Plan of Eating, if we find it useful.

After a while you may be amazed at how all the days that you take just one at a time suddenly and miraculously turn into weeks, months or years. You may wonder, for example, how *you* could possibly have managed to go two weeks, three months or seven years without a single compulsive bite, yet the answer is straightforward – we take one day at a time.

If you've been using a Plan of Eating consistently for a while and it no longer feels like something useful to you, you could always drop it. Just be watchful of your eating patterns after doing so and if you sense that you are slipping back into compulsions, review your notes, re-read this book and resume daily planning, if it serves you.

(You can find more detailed information on Trigger Lists, writing a Plan of Eating and more in my first book *How to go Raw for Weight Loss*.)

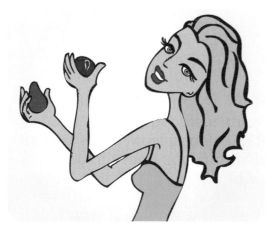

How a Plan of Eating Might Look...

Let's consider a sample Plan of Eating. '**Sadie**' is transitioning from being a 'cooked food vegetarian' into adopting a raw vegan lifestyle. She just started this new journey into eating high-raw three weeks ago. She intends to be 100% raw at some point, though for now she still enjoys eating a few cooked foods. The Vigour foods she has already discovered that she loves are avocados, sunflower seeds, walnuts, tomatoes and cherries. She has not long 'let go' of a compulsion for wheat spaghetti and rich tomato sauce; bread is also a major Trigger Food for her. Below is a sample daily Plan of Eating that she might use. *Remember* that this is *Sadie's* Plan. Everybody is different in terms of quantities, foods chosen and the number of meals in a day. Your Plan will be tailored to you. This is just to give you an idea...

A High-Raw Daily Food Plan:

Breakfast: one cereal bowl of raw muesli (apple, banana, sunflower seeds, pumpkin seeds, raisins, cinnamon, almond milk)

Snack: 1lb (500g) of cherries

Lunch: Three nori rolls stuffed with fresh vegetables, ginger and cooked brown rice

Snacks: 16oz (500ml) smoothie made with fruit and greens; handful of walnuts

Dinner: 16oz (500ml) green vegetable juice, followed by salad w/ avocado dressing & flax crackers

(N.B. It is of course recommended to drink water throughout the day too – preferably at least 3 to 4 quarts/litres daily. However, you need not include water in your written Plan, unless you feel it serves you to do so.) Again, you can read a lot more about Plans of Eating in my first book *How to Go Raw for Weight Loss.*

Planning: Civilisation or 'The Wild Way'?

Some people may look at the way others eat – perhaps an 'Animalistic Human' such as Anastasia, living 'wild' out in the Siberian forest (see page 32) – and feel resentment: '*She* doesn't make a Plan of Eating, so why should I?' Why, indeed? Certainly no-one is forcing you – it is a choice. Ask yourself this though: has what you've been doing until now brought you results that you felt good about? If not, to get different results we can start taking different actions. Making a Plan of Eating is a tried and tested way to turn your habits around.

Also, most of us live in a manner very far removed from the reality of someone like Anastasia (out in the forest) or tribal nomads. Yes, they don't make Food Plans; they also don't live disconnected from nature like most of us do, using money, formal education, motor vehicles or many of the other aspects of 'civilisation'. We live differently in almost every other regard yet may want to eat spontaneously, like they do. Isn't that interesting? The kind of societies we live in are *based* on structure – we plan our houses, our families, our cities, our activities, our working schedules...we live with calendars, budgets, deadlines, appointments and clocks...yet we don't want to plan our daily food intake. I am not suggesting that every person in a 'civilised' setting *ought* to be making a daily Plan of Eating, or that living with imposed structure is in any way ideal – far from it in fact. A Food Plan is simply a tool that *can* be used if you feel it might benefit your journey. I recommend at least giving it a try for a few days.

When someone like Anastasia makes food choices, there is no other *possibility* for her there in the Siberian forest than to eat simple, natural foods, straight from the Earth. In this sense, she might be considered truly blessed. There is nothing else *there* to choose, even if she wanted to (and I'm quite confident that she would not want to eat processed foods anyway). We, however, tend to live in very different environments. Our lifestyles are far from 'natural', with our concrete houses, cars, clothes, processed foods, office blocks, air conditioning, factories, stores and so on. When we try to spontaneously reach out for food, we encounter literally millions of products to choose from, many of which are *physiologically addictive*, remember. This in itself gives a new angle to the saying 'spoilt for choice'! Few of us in our modern societies regularly, if ever, go out and gather our foods by hand from nature. Instead, we have cupboards, freezers and fridges stacked with food. We have such abundance, right there, piled up in our kitchens: we're surrounded by it.

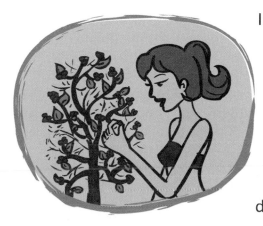

Imagine that today you only ate things that you foraged from your area. What would you be eating? Berries, flowers, greens, shoots, roots, nuts, maybe some mushrooms? Your choices would be significantly simpler and your quantities likely smaller. In our societies we are *deluged* by 'food' choices, very few of them raw or natural, let alone organic. This can feel overwhelming and is a 'recipe' for over-indulging.

It can be shocking to consider that there are now so many humans on Earth and so much land has been damaged (especially by modern farming) that we actually couldn't realistically sustain ourselves as a species if we *did* all try to go out and forage from now on. Our best alternative is to get educated about simpler ways of living – like eating raw – and ideally to start growing much of our own food, focusing on Permaculture principles, sprouting, growing microgreens and so on (see the Resources section for more info).

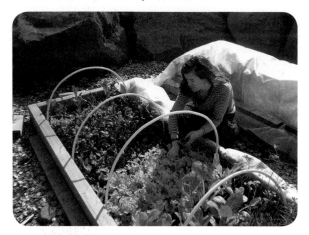

While Anastasia's way of eating looks spontaneous and 'free', if we look a little closer there is, of course, *some* kind of inherent structure to the way she eats. The forest she lives in is **full** of things to potentially consume. Yet not all of these things are 'food' for humans; indeed, many are poisonous to us. This **awareness** of what is 'food' in Anastasia's environment can be considered a template of understanding, passed down through the generations. We can think of it this way: just because you can put something in your mouth doesn't mean it's a real food for us (and that applies wherever you are – forest or city). In the forest, the choices of foods have been narrowed and defined over the years by both experience and intuition, into a kind of 'integrated intelligence'. This 'intelligence in context' has been undisturbed for centuries, especially in terms of non-exposure to commercial/non-local alternatives.

In contrast, we in the West might be thought of as having experienced a severe disruption in the chain of passing on such information in *our* societies, as well as ongoing re-arrangements of our physical food-bearing landscape. When we encounter the confusing plethora of things presented as food in our societies, we face attempting to decipher for *ourselves* what is truly nourishing, based on educated discernment, rather than a more innate wisdom. We might think of these efforts to make sense of our food landscape and to choose foods that are naturally and truly nourishing like 'the reconciliation after the divorce'. We've been cut off from simpler choices for a long time, yet we can do our best to make sense of things, based on the information that we can access. Currently, we are fortunate that there is a renaissance of understanding about what is truly nourishing and we can all tap into this through individuals, groups, books, the internet and so on.

Returning to the idea of making a Plan of Eating, consider that we are accustomed to structure in most areas of our lives – we trust it and rely on it. Then, when we try to eat spontaneously, without discernment, it can all end in circles of self-destruction. If we were living out in the wild, like Anastasia, then our food choices would of course be very different and having a Food Plan would likely become rapidly obsolete. As it is, if we are called to continue living in the 'modern' world, it truly can be a relief to add in structure around our food choices, along with all the other structures in our lives. Otherwise, it seems all too easy to reach out for the usual Trigger foods we're addicted to – physiologically and emotionally.

Our current societal infrastructure is not yet set up to support very easy access to raw foods. It's usually much easier to find toxic, unnatural foods that reflect our 'unnatural' lifestyles. Without a structured Plan to help us have available the foods we choose, it's very easy to think to ourselves, 'Well, I'll just *have* to grab this slice of pizza, since there's nothing else here to eat...'

Saucy Salvation

A great tip for 'being prepared' as a raw foodie is to regularly make up big batches of some kind of yummy raw sauce. This might be a basil pesto, a tomato sauce, a creamy cashew dip or whatever you enjoy. Keep this sauce on hand in your fridge, to use as and when required. You might use it as a sauce for (raw) pasta, a salad dressing, a spread for flax crackers, a dip for crudités and so on. You can thin it down with more liquid or thicken it up with ground flax/chia. This is a very simple, quick, versatile way to 'stay in the game', rather than thinking, 'There's nothing here to eat, so I'm going to eat these chips instead'.

We can avert this pattern as raw foodists if we take a little time to plan what we would like to eat each day and are sure to **be prepared**, as we go about our day, in places where raw foods may not yet be easily available.

This might all come over as a little extreme, as though you have the choice to *either* live in the wild and eat naturally from food sources as you find them, OR to live in a 'civilised' world and plan your meals. In practice though, it doesn't have to be one choice or the other – there is a middle ground. Find your own formula that supports you in carrying through your positive intent. Particularly when you are first ringing in your raw changes, a clear Plan is invaluable. If you take care to have the foods you desire on hand, being in areas where raw foods aren't readily available is not an issue. As always, **the choice is yours** as to whether or not you use this tool. I, for one, can definitely understand feeling resistance to it, as you'll see here:

I was very resistant about making a Plan of Eating in the beginning. I thought stubbornly, 'I don't need some tedious daily list of what to eat'. I found the idea of deciding beforehand exactly what I was going to eat that day deeply dull and restrictive.

*However, I saw that what I **had** been doing wasn't serving me, so, I dropped my shield of pride and wrote my first daily Plan. One day at a time, I wrote my Plan, shared it with another and stuck to it. When I walked past stands handing out free samples in supermarkets, I reminded myself that I'd not put that free sample of cake on my food list today and walked on. When I encountered luxurious buffets of delicious raw foods at potlucks, I reminded myself of my commitment to eat just one plate of food and nothing more, and so on. Slowly, slowly I began to build trust in myself again as I followed my Food Plan, day by day. Gone were the broken 'I'll just eat one of these...' promises, replaced with a simple, practical Plan. Using a Plan of Eating frees up my time and energy and brings me serenity and new joy. I also find that sharing my daily intake through my online e-journal (http://rawreform.blogspot. com) helps me enormously to stay 'accountable' to myself and monitor my intake.*

A New Life Awaits

If you have followed the guidance given here and done the three simple writing tasks above - the History Review, Trigger/Vigour Lists and Plan of Eating - you have formed a solid base for breaking any addictive patterns with food. If you 'slithered past' doing the writing, I strongly suggest that you head on back and give yourself the gift of writing these invaluable notes. Scoot back up to pages 78-84.

You can refer back to your writing whenever you feel the need. Instead of going on some standard diet or rushing into going raw without any preparation, you can do a little foundation work now to create focus and awareness of where you're coming from and where you want to go. You can then get on with your new lifestyle. It is a very grounded approach.

Real transformation work to break addictive patterns is about *action*, not knowledge. You can read and learn lots of things about how to manage emotional attachments, compulsive overeating or being raw, yet without actually putting anything into *action*, without making and following a Plan, that knowledge is worth very little. Stay in action, or you might head into destruction.

So now it's time to relinquish the foods and patterns that have not been serving your health. Follow the tasks outlined here to open a doorway to a new and solid lifestyle of radiant healthy living – enjoy!

Intro to Emotional Detox

In the last few sections, we've been learning all about the connections between our *emotions* and *eating*, including cravings, addictions and personal patterns – some of which are compulsive and unsupportive of vibrant health. We've also worked through a three-step plan to help shift those patterns and lovingly laid out our Optimal Vision for our lives (...haven't we...?).

We've seen how food can be used as one way to suppress and avoid real emotional connections. We realise that we want to experience positive shifts, leaving those old patterns behind. Now we can delve deeper into the 'emotional detox' – what does that mean? What will come up? What will we be releasing?

Before we begin exploring the details of emotional release, I think it's important to note that *emotional* detox follows the same kind of path as *physical* detox. For this reason, it is advisable to take it slowly.

We did not get into a tangled emotional web overnight and it would be pretty intense to try to untangle all of our emotional issues overnight too. Most people have a lot to release and this takes time. If we have a lot of re-programming to do, it's likely to take a while to shift out of our old patterns and habits into a new routine.

Slowly, slowly, one day at a time, we can transform our patterns if we keep making positive choices. We are not only dealing with releasing the *old* stored 'negative' emotions, we are also learning to handle the emotions that come up for us now in a more positive way.

> *"Health is not a state to aim for, but a process*
> *to be continuously involved in."*
> *--Paul Benson*

What Is It Like to Go Through Emotional Detox?

Ultimately, it's all good news...

As we start to heal, our skewed emotional connections with food begin to shift. We **stop using food as a crutch** – we feel really alive rather than doped up on our 'drug' of choice. We begin to re-orientate towards eating to enhance health, joyful living and our communion with the Divine. As what we eat ceases to be the most important thing to us, life becomes fuller and more beautiful. Our emotions feel *raw*, just like our bodies. At first we might feel 'wide open' or exposed as we learn to identify and feel our feelings rather than suppress them. We are no longer hiding behind food. It may all feel very unfamiliar. Yet as we stay with it, we see that our limiting thoughts dissolve. It feels progressively easier to be healthy and happy. We might even start to share our story with others and inspire them to make shifts. Incidentally, it can be a very wise move to warn family, friends and loved-ones as you go into this process that you might be a little wobbly emotionally for the first few weeks or so. Preparing people in this way can make a real difference in the event that you find yourself 'bouncing off the walls' with emotional output.

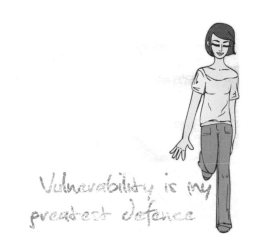

Vulnerability is my greatest defence

Negativity and **blocked energies** are stored in excess fat. When we start to put more live foods into our bodies, toxins and energies leave those 'deadened' places and releasing is activated on many levels. As we release the extra physical weight, the blocked energies stored within it naturally begin to dis-engage and we can let go of all those long-since trapped negative feelings like self-loathing, anger, fear, loneliness, guilt, depression and so on. This is an incredible process, yet one that people frequently find scary to even contemplate, let alone experience. This trepidation is one reason why many revert to their old patterns and regain weight after releasing it: the emotional detox just feels like too much to handle. However if we actively work through the emotional blockages, our life can shift to a space where everything, including our relationship with food, becomes more loving and joyous.

At the same time as releasing *old* bottled-up emotions, our day-to-day emotions can also be seen in terms of a **continuous flow**. Feelings *will* inevitably come up for us around things, as feelings do.

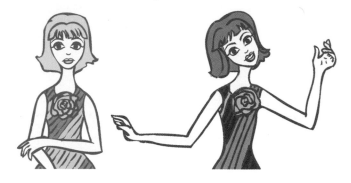

If we express our feelings rather than hold them in, the easier it is all around. Suppressing and holding onto our feelings can create inner toxicity and detrimentally affect our outlook and relationships. (We'll take a more detailed look into healthy ways to express emotions on the following pages.)

You may find that your emotions at times feel somewhat 'wild' – maybe you're infused with exuberance, constantly crying, or experiencing confusion. As we now know, **emotions come and go**, just like food cravings. When we simply allow our feelings to be what they are rather than trying to hide or stifle them, they pass *so* much faster.

As things are released, you may feel great – you may also feel very uncomfortable. If you feel the latter, the good news is that this too shall pass (whether you eat in response to it or not).

Ever wondered why an unpleasant emotion seems to lurch up 'out of the blue'? You may find, for example, that you are suddenly filled with huge resentment towards an ex-partner whom you haven't thought about for years. If you start to examine your feelings around this, you might remember that during this relationship you often felt unattractive/rejected and would eat to comfort yourself. Now, as your body is releasing those old accumulated fat deposits from those days, those suppressed emotions come up and out, too... Remind yourself regularly that it is OK to feel all your feelings – whatever they are, they are valid and valuable parts of you that come and *go* in natural rhythms.

Trying to stop your pain by ignoring or denying feelings simply re-enforces emotional blocks and tension, as well as setting you up for relapse. So, quite simply, don't do it. Acknowledge your feelings, identify them, and allow them to move through... If you feel you need to, share your feelings with safe people and move on.

Tuning In

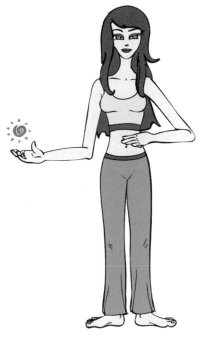

I recommend getting into the practice of tuning into *where* in your body tension is coming from whenever you feel uncomfortable. On the surface you might be in a traffic jam, or dealing with someone you feel annoyed by or some other similar situation – and you choose to 'blame' this for your tension. Try to look beyond this superficial tension, however. There is almost always something deeper that is unsettling your being. What is the real source of your tension; where is it located?

Frequently, you'll discover that there is a sense of blocked energy around your third chakra (the solar plexus area, about three fingers' width above the belly button). If you really concentrate your focus on that area, get honest, breathe deeply into it and try to relax, you may start to tune into the underlying source of your frustrations. Trust any images/feelings that come up – if you're in a traffic jam though, pay attention to your driving too!

Tension felt in the solar plexus chakra is usually concerned with issues you believe that you have no control over. You might realise, for instance, that actually you don't enjoy your job and feel powerless to make necessary changes. Or you may find yourself aware of tension in your marriage. Tension most often stems from the fact that in some way you are living in fear about something. This may be fear of abandonment, fears about economic security, fear of illness and so on. All of these anxieties can be shifted significantly by using some of the tips shared in this book and stepping away from operating from fear, into fully embodying the love that we are.

It may be that a number of 'big' issues all seem to bubble up for you at the same time. No need to feel overwhelmed. You *can work* through anything that comes up for you. The situation is far from 'hopeless'. Just take gentle note of your feelings in the moment and be glad of the awareness. The point of this exercise is to realise that superficial incidents like getting annoyed with a checkout clerk, freaking out because your bag breaks and so on are all indicative of an underlying absence of serenity. None are disastrous events in themselves – however, they can *feel* like 'the straw that broke the camel's back' if your inner sense of peace is not well established. If this sounds familiar, recognise that there is likely a deeper tension in you, the resolution of which can help you fall into happier alignment within yourself and with all around you.

What Are 'Chakras'?

Most people are aware that there are different subtle energy circuits that run through the body (for example, those tapped into during acupuncture). The chakra system can be thought of as a series of swirling, dynamic vortexes in the body – 'wheels of light' – through which energy flows. There are seven main centres in our torsos. They run from the base/root chakra, located near our seat bones (red), up through the lower and upper abdomen, the heart space, throat, third eye, then crown chakra (violet). Each chakra relates to certain aspects of our lives and personalities. In many people, one or more of the chakra channels is out of balance, or blocked, which can interrupt energy flow. Awakening the chakras and bringing them into balanced alignment with each other can rapidly assist our healing. For more details, please look into healer Martin Brofman's work using chakras: http://www.healer.ch/Chakras-e.html.

Whenever you have an emotionally charged experience, breathe in deeply, embrace the release without judgement, forgive and send love to both yourself and all those involved. It may feel quite odd and unfamiliar at first to approach your emotions in this way. It may take courage, patience and commitment to stay with the process, especially if those around you are not moving into healing in the same way as you. I thoroughly recommend getting support for this process: speak to others who have been through similar experiences, join a support group, go on a retreat somewhere where it feels 'safe' to release pent-up emotions and so on. The Guidance section below provides a long list of practical suggestions for handling the emotional detox.

Socially, going raw can have its challenges in the beginning. We don't always have the benefit of immediate understanding and acceptance from those around us when we choose to make changes in our life. We may expe-

rience shaming, criticism and anxiety about the direction we are moving in. To some people, the raw lifestyle can even seem threatening.

Going raw usually involves facing food issues and making large shifts in a person's life. If you dive in and experience this, it might feel 'threatening' to others around you, showing them that they could possibly do this too. This may be something they are not ready or willing to experience and social rifts can form as a result. Still, as you now know, you are not alone. There are plenty of resources, people and tools to help you on your way, as outlined here. Raw communities are constantly expanding as more people become aware and active in transforming their health – see the Resources section for contacts.

As we progress with emotional detox, it can feel like our emotions get more and **more sensitive**, so keep this in your awareness. This follows a similar pattern to the physical detox that our bodies experience. The longer someone is raw, the cleaner and more sensitive the physical body becomes. If we then eat some non-raw processed foods, we can end up in a lot of pain.

(See my partner Matt Monarch's landmark book *Raw Success* for in-depth details on the *physical* aspects of sensitivities and success with a raw lifestyle in the long-run).

This 'increasing sensitivity' pattern can be mirrored with our emotions. The longer one is raw, the more the *emotional* field becomes increasingly 'clean' and vibrant too, filled with love, joy, sincerity and similar feelings. We seek true heart connections with others and balance. If we then go into a very negative-feeling space, it can feel quite drastic and caustic, as we've become so accustomed to living in a joyous state. Even a small imbalance from that place of deep, loving acceptance can feel very disruptive, as it's such a stark contrast from the happiness you've been experiencing. You might feel like you're 'spinning out' on an undesirable trajectory from the space you were enjoying and that everything feels a bit out of control and unpleasant.

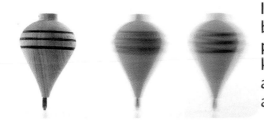

I like to use the analogy of a very delicate, beautiful spinning top that spins in perpetual graceful motion. If it gets slightly knocked, however, it crashes and spins out across the room, bashing into everything around it, until it is gently picked up and set in motion again. These kinds of emotional 'crash' experiences can definitely be taken as warning signals that your thoughts have been heading in a other-than-optimal direction for your ultimate well-being. At the same time, it is important to remember that, like all feelings, this too shall pass. Re-orientate your focus if you feel you have slipped off track. Simply pick up your 'spinning top', give it a twirl and cruise onwards at a gentler pace...

In the process of emotional detox and the return to our true selves, we come to understand that regardless of what appears to be unfolding around us, we can be happy in every moment if we choose to be. Every experience is an opportunity. Regardless of the weather, the work we're engaged in, the personalities we encounter in any given day, we can feel joy and serenity, if that is our choice. Attitude is everything – and it is completely under our control. I can often be heard saying, *'It's all OK if we say it is'*. I truly believe that. Our experience in any situation hinges on how we feel. If we *choose* to feel good, give love into the situation and breathe deeply, we can get through anything. As Abraham Lincoln succinctly put it: 'Most folks are about as happy as they make up their minds to be.'

The book *Alcoholics Anonymous* contains a list of particularly inspiring 'promises' for those recovering from addictions. They can be applied to recovery from any addiction and are as follows:

- We are going to know a new freedom and a new happiness.
- We will not regret the past nor wish to shut the door on it.
- We will comprehend the word 'serenity' and we will know peace.
- No matter how far down the scale we have gone, we will see how our experience can benefit others.
- That feeling of uselessness and self-pity will disappear.
- We will lose interest in selfish things and gain interest in our fellows.
- Self-seeking will slip away.
- Our whole attitude and outlook upon life will change.
- Fear of people and of economic insecurity will leave us.
- We will intuitively know how to handle situations that used to baffle us.
- We will suddenly realise that God is doing for us what we could not do for ourselves.
- Are these extravagant promises? We think not.
- They are being fulfilled among us - sometimes quickly, sometimes slowly.
- They will always materialise if we work for them.

I hope that you find motivation and inspiration for your own transformation from reading these 'promises'.

Blockages to Healing

Perverse though it may sound, many people truly seem afraid to be healthy, energetic and lively. They are afraid to heal. If they lose their excess weight, heal their emotional wounds, stop living life as a 'victim'...what then? What will there be to complain about? How will they get attention? What will there be to hide behind? What will happen if, for example, their cholesterol is suddenly fine and there are no medical statistics to grumble about? In a sense, such people identify very strongly with their illnesses, even seeming to confuse the sickness with who they really are, at core.

People may deny this attachment at a conscious level, yet a simple observation of their behaviour will likely reveal otherwise. They appear to relish the details of how much medicine they are taking, how their appointments with their doctor went, the 'suffering' they experience as a result of their condition and so on. There is massive attachment at play here, clearly seen, even on a visual level, in those who are overweight/obese. The excess fat is a literal protective layer – a buffer against the world, within which to hide. This toxic layer of false safety can be used as a reason (conscious or otherwise) to sidestep shining to one's full potential. As a result of living inside this fat layer we may:

*procrastinate work projects, avoiding feeling successful
*perpetuate self-pity
*feel very negative about life, rejected/unsupported – worry a lot
*live like control freaks – especially where food is concerned
*feel like food is our only true, reliable friend
*avoid intimacy/romance/sex
*numb ourselves from responsibility and our true life path
*feel lonely/misunderstood and use food to alleviate that pain
*stay in a victim position, or angry with the world
*maintain co-dependent relationships, fearing possible rejection/jealousy if we change (e.g. in a family where being overweight is the norm.)

However, major shifts can potentially happen when we begin to shine the torchlight of consciousness on our relationship with food, divinity and ourselves. We are no longer easily able to live in denial about our issues. This is where choosing to see ourselves and to behave as 'Active Transformers' really comes in.

We have learned that many of us try to avoid facing our issues, addictions or fears, yet this very avoidance keeps us trapped in vicious circles of denial and suppressed emotions, creating even more issues. Choose instead to deal with your challenges and the truth of your patterns head-on. Using the strategy of 'dealing with the worst first' is a great help; after getting the biggest issues in your head straightened out, the rest will seem easy in comparison.

This popular piece of writing by Marianne Williamson on the theme of removing blocks in our lives became especially well-known after Nelson Mandela quoted it during his inauguration speech in 1994. It is a great inspiration for transforming fears and becoming who you are here to be:

Our deepest fear is not that we are inadequate.
Our deepest fear is that we are powerful beyond measure.
It is our light, not our darkness that most frightens us.
We ask ourselves, "Who am I to be brilliant, gorgeous, talented, fabulous?"
Actually, who are you not to be?
You are a child of God.
Your playing small does not serve the world.
There is nothing enlightened about shrinking so that other people won't feel insecure around you.
We are all meant to shine, as children do.
We were born to make manifest the glory of God that is within us. It's not just in some of us; it's in everyone.
And as we let our own light shine, we unconsciously give other people permission to do the same.
As we are liberated from our own fear, our presence automatically liberates others.

Taking a Closer Look

We now know that, although the raw food lifestyle is a great ally in releasing addictions and embracing radiant health, it's a challenge to heal oneself with *just* raw food. We could use another ally in this process: a *broader* understanding of our emotions and patterns, with supportive tools to help transform these areas. It's time to think about the emotional matters *beyond the food…*

In order for emotional healing to take place, there are certain common core issues that addicts can benefit from addressing. Self-help author Charles L. Whitfield writes lucidly about these. For example, it's important to be able to grieve for that which we have lost/never had and also to 'be real' – be who we really are rather than presenting ourselves as we think others want to see us. We can learn to identify and express our feelings. We can stop neglecting our own needs, tolerating inappropriate behaviour or being overly responsible for others. We can examine our low self-esteem, control and trust issues and all-or-nothing thinking. We can face our fear of abandonment, difficulty handling conflict and our issues with giving and receiving love.

This is no small order and it is beyond the scope of this book to go into extensive detail on this topic (though we certainly do explore these issues to an extent and provide practical suggestions in the Guidance section). We are talking about trying to un-numb ourselves from an emotional coma and unravel a *lifetime* of learned behaviour, which is *essential* to keep us out of overeating and other compulsions. These are the **core issues** that are intertwined with our addictive behaviour.

In the next few pages, before we launch into the Guidance section, we'll be looking a little more closely at these deeper emotional issues and patterns that we might be living with and potentially wanting to release. We'll be enquiring into ten key areas we may want to address for release work, including 'inner child' issues, shaming, defences, boundaries and co-dependency. We are aiming for balance in our emotional health.

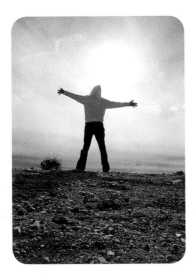

Taking a look at these 'deeper' matters may help us get back in touch with our *true* emotions and feelings, which in turn can help us relate more easily to ourselves as well as others. Our whole lives take on fresh meaning and direction as we uncover and share who we *really* are. Also, the more we know about our selves and patterns, the less likely it is that we'll turn back to our old addictions as coping mechanisms.

> One of the easiest ways to start to reconnect and reawaken to our true selves is simply to pay attention to our feelings...

Feeling the Feelings

Our feelings guide us on our life paths and no feeling is 'wrong'. Every feeling – happy, angry, sad, worried, lonely – is a valuable and valid part of us. As we transform, we learn to accept and value our feelings exactly as they are, without trying to deny them, cover them up or feeling shame about them. Face your feelings, experience them and let them pass. Feelings, like cravings, come and go rather quickly, yet if we are not used to that process it can seem intense, especially in the early stages of transformation.

The first step in learning to cope with your feelings is to simply be *aware* of them. Once you know what you're dealing with, you begin to have choices about how to act on those feelings to dissolve any old patterns. Let's take a look at some key feelings that tend to come up during transformation and our behaviour connected to them:

- ANGER. Many of us received no modelling on how to process anger in a healthy way. It is important here to remember the difference between *feeling* angry and *acting* on it. We don't have to act violently or abusively if we feel angry; no-one has to get hurt. A healthy way to learn to deal with anger is simply to talk about it, identify it and resolve the feelings beneath it. Anger nearly always stems from fear of some kind. Talk things through, rather than acting out, and choose not to engage in blaming, sarcasm and name-calling. For many, it is also important to realise that others won't abandon us if we say we're angry. We are just being honest about our feelings and clearing the air.

- SHAME. If we were shamed or ridiculed for our feelings and needs as children, we will often feel uneasy and even disgusted with ourselves in transformation when we begin to reconnect to these parts of ourselves. Such 'toxic' shaming is one of the most potentially damaging experiences we can undergo during development. We may now experience great difficulty sharing our needs and feelings with others. We may live in a state of toxic shame, being very self-critical, feeling flawed and unworthy. It is important therefore to learn to **value**

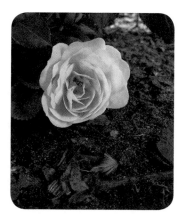

ourselves, our feelings and needs as important and to find supportive, non-shaming people with whom to share.

- LONELINESS. Food addicts are often very isolated from others - excess food appears to us as a lifeline. When we stop eating those foods, our sense of loneliness and abandonment can therefore greatly deepen because we are essentially letting go of what feels like the most important relationship in our lives. Hence it is all the more important to begin at this time to build a supportive network around yourself of 'safe' people. It is OK to say that you feel lonely – you do not have to be alone.

- GRIEF. As well as loneliness, when we 'put down' the excess food, we often experience a real sense of loss. This is a grief reaction from losing an important relationship and we may experience confusion, emptiness, sadness, fear, doubts and preoccupation with thinking of the loss. This is all quite normal and is also the time when your addicted mind is likely to suggest things like 'it's OK to just have one piece of this, you're not *that* addicted'. Be aware that grief is a **process**, usually following this pattern: denial and isolation, anger, bargaining ('maybe just one is OK'), sadness over the loss, letting go and then acceptance. Be aware of where you are in this process. Don't fight the feelings and give yourself time to grieve the loss.

- ASSERTIVENESS. Many of us have very cloudy, co-dependent boundaries with others. We don't know how to say 'no' when we want to, we avoid conflict at all costs and do not seek healthy respect for our boundaries. In recovery we can learn to be assertive, to stand up for our side of things. This might feel scary, but it does not have to be painful for anyone. We can feel assertive without being *aggressive* by simply communicating honestly and openly about our needs and feelings, rather than hiding them away.

- FEAR. Any changes, even positive ones, can conjure fear and anxiety. During recovery we have many changes to face, which can result in a lot of fear. Symptoms of anxiety such as a racing heart, shakiness, tension, irritability and excessive worry are common. Many of us have had no healthy modelling of how to attend to fear. We can now learn that feeling scared does not have to mean something bad will happen. It is OK to feel afraid - if we embrace the fear and let it pass, we will find peace on the other side.

When feelings come up for you, do your best to *immediately* go 'full-thrust' into the experience. In that way, the feeling doesn't block and stagnate for later and there is a greater chance that difficult emotions will clear rapidly and authentically.

We can learn to identify and share our emotions, especially in a supportive environment where we feel free to express ourselves; '12 Step' groups are particularly good for such sharing. Seek out 'safe' people who genuinely listen to you, are emotionally available, non-shaming, non-judgemental, give you healthy validation and do not push advice on what you 'should' or 'must' do or feel. If we were never supported to freely express our feelings as children, we have a lot to re-learn as adults. Try to practice patience and understanding with yourself – not criticism – during this important learning process.

What is '12 Step' Work?

The 12 Step programme of recovery is a highly respected, central resource for people in recovery. This rewarding programme includes many different aspects – fellowship groups, meetings, literature, 'sponsorship' from others in recovery, online resources and occasional retreats, to name a few. The programme offers a non-pushy, dynamic and powerful space for recovery that has helped transform the lives of millions.

The original 12 Step programme was that of Alcoholics Anonymous (AA), which started in Ohio, USA, in June 1935. It is a spiritual programme of recovery that provides a highly effective, 24/7 system of support and communication for alcoholics. These days there are many other 12 Step recovery programmes, covering many different addictions, all of which are based on the original 12 Steps and traditions of AA and promote honesty and spirituality. It is not a 'religious' programme - members may be from any religious background or none at all. It is based on acceptance of spiritual values that everyone is free to interpret as they choose. Other 12 Step fellowships include Narcotics Anonymous, Debtors Anonymous, Gamblers Anonymous, Co-Dependents Anonymous and of course, Overeaters Anonymous.

As the root of all addictions is basically the same - a loss of connection to our true selves – the materials and concepts used in the original AA programme can be easily used or adapted by other 12 Step fellowships. The central piece of literature in AA – *Alcoholics Anonymous* or '*The Big Book*', as it is affectionately known – is often used as the main recovery tool in other 12 Step fellowships too. The 12 Steps for recovery are based on spiritual wisdom and the experiences of others who have successfully used this approach to transform their lives. The simple truth is that this programme works – millions of 12-Steppers around the world lead happier, more productive lives, freed from compulsive behaviour, as a result of working this programme. You can find out more about 12 Step groups from links in the Resources section.

Phases of depression can also occur while you are undergoing big shifts in recovery, so be on the lookout for this. Depression is typically characterised by abnormally intense and prolonged feelings of sadness, panic, fear, anger or rage, as well as long periods of 'doom and gloom', sarcasm and negative perspectives. It is important to treat depression, so if you believe you may be depressed, do seek natural healing methods, with guidance from an experienced alternative health care professional if you choose.

Releasing

In the next section, we consider further what kind of issues might come up for us during detox. We will then delve into the Guidance section, which offers sixty effective ways to handle our emotions constructively.

What Might You Be Looking to Release?

We can think of human beings as conglomerations of habits and patterns. Some of those patterns are beneficial; many of them may no longer serve our optimal health and well-being. Instead, these patterns drain our energy and are strongly intertwined with any addictions we may experience, such as overeating. As we now know, it's very beneficial to take a good look at our emotional patterns and how they developed, then – once we have self-awareness – begin to make choices about how to dismantle any destructive cycles.

Most of these patterns are learned in childhood and are part of our family structures. They are deeply entrenched. Indeed, compliance with some of them may have felt essential for our *survival* as youngsters. It may feel almost taboo to acknowledge some of these patterns in ourselves. Our loyalty to our family structure may also blind us so much that even now, as adults, we are reluctant to view these patterns objectively, perhaps even openly denying that they persist. I thoroughly encourage you to read through the following list with your heart and mind open. Approach this task with *absolute honesty* and as much objectivity as you can muster.

Ten Things to Consider Releasing:

'Negative' Thinking

Just as most of us didn't grow up eating fresh raw food - something we may now consider optimal nutrition – we also didn't necessarily grow up with positive thinking/thought patterns/support as the norm. Our childhood may have been characterised by environments where 'negativity', judgement, sarcasm, criticism, blaming, shaming, exaggeration, self-pity, anxiety, fear and even depression prevailed. As children, we seek acceptance by those around us, so we absorb those other-than-optimal ways of thinking and being into our own patterns, most likely without question. After years and years of practice, these patterns are so assimilated that they are virtually un-conscious. When we take an honest look at how we view the world, we might feel truly *entrenched* in these negative thought processes. When we go raw or start seeking transformation in our lives, these 'lower-vibration' thoughts and feelings start jarring against our new highest vision for ourselves of how we'd love to be living.

As you experience the restructuring that physical and emotional transforma-tion brings, old thought patterns will still continue to 'speak' to you, just as old food cravings will come and go. Remember that in every moment, you have a choice. You are the director of the show. The more often you choose to focus on the positive aspects of your experiences, the more refined you will become at noticing negative thought patterns and stepping away from them, while you simultaneously generate and attract increasing amounts of positivity.

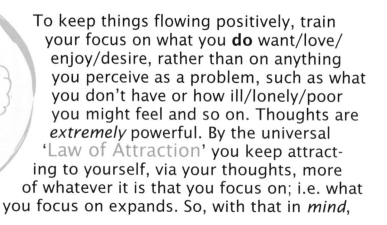

To keep things flowing positively, train your focus on what you **do** want/love/ enjoy/desire, rather than on anything you perceive as a problem, such as what you don't have or how ill/lonely/poor you might feel and so on. Thoughts are *extremely* powerful. By the universal 'Law of Attraction' you keep attract-ing to yourself, via your thoughts, more of whatever it is that you focus on; i.e. what you focus on expands. So, with that in *mind*,

A Secret Smile…

Sometimes our body language can reveal interesting things about our patterns. For example, have you noticed that some people actually *smile* as they talk about perceived 'difficulties' in their lives? Sometimes of course, this appears as the gentle smile of someone who is aware that ultimately, all is well, whatever appears to be happening on the surface. More frequently, though, this pattern seems to arise in those who tend to focus on 'issues/problems' in life – e.g. 'Did I tell you, Uncle Billy's going in for a knee operation again?'; 'The service at that restaurant was awful – the waitress was so rude'; or 'I told them that would happen – they never listen to me' and so on. Although the topic is something that might usually be thought of as unfortunate/unpleasant, the speaker is smiling. There is a sense that they actually enjoy focusing on these aspects of life or even delight in it in some way. They might dwell on details and repeat such stories often. What might be behind that smile? My feeling is that usually, focusing on 'the negative' is a life-long pattern for such speakers and it is what feels comfortable to them. In contrast, speaking about inspiring, uplifting, exciting, expansive ideas and projects might seem alien and perhaps even scary to someone whose reality until now has been mainly shaped by 'negative' imprinting.

Be aware of your *own* facial expressions in the coming days as you speak. Do you notice yourself smiling if you speak about 'difficulties'? Does this seem peculiar to you? What do you think might underlie this pattern?

I recognised this pattern in *myself* only when it was pointed out to me one day by a friend. I was relaying a story I'd told many times before of how challenging my relationship had been with an ex-partner. My friend listened as I told this 'tale of woe' then asked me why I'd had a slight smile on my face the whole time I spoke. What was 'in it' for me to keep repeating this story? How was this serving me? This was a real moment of clarity for me and helped me to move on and let go of that pattern.

This is not to suggest, however, that we all ought to look morose, tearful or distraught whenever we relay other-than-fabulous information. It is simply a pattern that *can* be observed and might reveal some interesting insights, if we are willing to explore…

what would you prefer to keep drawing unto yourself? Positive, enriching, glowing experiences, or mundane, depressing, energy-draining situations? It's all a choice.

Things can be a little slow to materialise here in the physical world. We might think of it this way: tomorrow is created by your thoughts today. *Today* is a result of your thinking yesterday. As you were going about your day yesterday, you were pre-paving your path for your experiences today. How did it work out for you? Are you having an outstanding time **today**? If not, what adjustments do you think you might be able to make today in your thought patterns to create a more joyful tomorrow (let alone a more uplifting present moment)?

World-renowned motivational speaker Anthony Robbins has a great movie analogy he uses to help people shift their focus. Have you ever seen a movie you really didn't enjoy? Would you then choose to watch that film over and over and *over* again? Probably not, right? Yet that is what so many of us do inside our head, day-in-day-out, dwelling on the past, re-living old angst, going round in circles of self-pity and misery. Is it time, perhaps, to put on a new movie...?

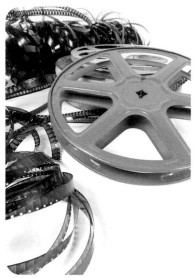

What do you want to experience? Where is your focus? Do you focus on your joy, your love? Or on how difficult things are and unlikely to work out? Where are your thoughts leading you? Let me be clear: this does not mean being 'unrealistic' about issues that may arise for you. We all experience challenges in life. Just remember to keep your outlook light. Try viewing your experiences here on Earth as a game, aware that you are choosing every experience you have. So, with that considered, are you going to choose to enjoy your time here or be in misery? The choice is absolutely yours, in every moment.

> *"Everything can be taken from a man but one thing; the last of the human freedoms - to choose one's attitude in any given set of circumstances, to choose one's own way."*
> *--Viktor Frankl*

Remember your Optimal Vision for your life? It helps to read it aloud to yourself sometimes as a reaffirming download and reminder. Why not take it out now and give it a read-through out loud, perhaps even polishing any parts that could be a bit more shiny?

Sometimes it may seem there is so much to undo from our past patterns that we feel exhausted by it, yet it may just be that we are unaware of how to draw in energy to support this process. Remember that it isn't a 'job lot' to be sorted out in one go, but rather something to gently unfold, bit by bit. I recommend applying some of the tips shared in the Guidance section below.

How I Embraced Positive Thinking...

I guess you could say that I learned about the power of positive thinking the 'tough way' - through personal experience. Many years ago, I began to pay attention to my communication with Spirit, listening and watching for 'clues'. I began to notice patterns, such as, if I was walking along and thinking critical thoughts about myself or others, I'd often find that I'd suddenly trip over. I came to see this as a **co-creation** *of my spirit, my physical body and the Universe, all working together to nudge me into remembering that those kinds of thoughts do not positively serve anyone. I would thank Spirit for the 'reminder' and withdraw my energy from such thoughts, moving to a more positive focus instead. This kind of pattern resonated through every aspect of my life. For example, if I was playing a board game and got into a headspace where I felt very competitive and determined to 'beat' the other person, based on satisfying my ego, the energy would seem to instantly move, making my position in the game less secure. If I was willing to let go, however and move back into a neutral space, there was still a chance that I might 'win' the game, but not from an ego space. The value of positive, open, loving thoughts was a big concept for me to absorb and I would sometimes get injured along the way - literally. I learned swiftly to avoid negative thought spaces when cutting things with knives. I learned that my being would make use of whatever was available in the situation and if a knife was what was at hand, then that's what was used...eeeeeek! Events like these helped me to learn quickly the value of thinking positively, at all times... These days, the vast majority of my thoughts are positive, joyous and loving and I am very grateful for the transformation. The more positive and loving my thoughts, the more joy and happy 'synchronicities' are attracted into my life. I'm sure my toes and fingers are all grateful too, though perhaps not my quietened 'ego'.*

For example, taking a course based around healing/positive patterns near the beginning of your transformation is likely to be *very* useful, as well as finding a support network, reading inspirational books and so on. Do whatever it takes to keep up your motivation and inspiration for a more positive outlook.

"All animals except man know that the principal business of life is to enjoy it."
--Samuel Butler

The Wounded Inner Child

This concept features regularly in self-help work. Childhood is a critical time for the development of a healthy individual, a time when patterns we learn from our caregivers are absorbed. If we do not receive genuine unconditional love, mirroring and acceptance for who we are as children, this leaves us prone to a lifetime of low self-esteem and denial of our own feelings. The kind of damaging messages we may have received directly or indirectly as children include:

- Don't cry – you have no reason to be upset.
- You should not be angry.
- Don't upset your mother or father.
- Don't be unhappy – we want to see you smiling.
- Don't disappoint us – we do so much for you.

The beautiful, loving, open, vulnerable child within us 'freezes' when we are not accepted for who we are, unconditionally. The full range of feelings that we start off with as children becomes gradually numbed down when we do not see those feelings expressed by others and so perceive them as unacceptable. We are thus not raised to identify and express our feelings in a healthy way.

By undertaking committed transformation work on the emotional and spiritual levels as adults, we can reconnect to our wounded child within, providing for *ourselves* the unconditional love, security and acceptance that we may not have received as children. It is important to note here that the aim of undertaking such 'inner child' work is not to find someone or something else to *blame* for our situation – far from it. Rather, we simply aim to get an honest overview of what happened during our emotional development to begin to have choices about dissolving unsupportive patterns.

The book *Homecoming* by John Bradshaw is a wonderful resource to start addressing 'Inner Child' issues - see page 213 for more details.

Roles

Many of us assume roles to cover over feelings of inadequacy, such as 'super-achiever', 'nice guy', 'people-pleaser' or 'joker', which provide a mask to hide behind, smothering our true feelings. We usually develop these roles from a young age if we do not receive mirroring for our *true* selves. Roles are coping mechanisms for getting acceptance in whichever way we can. People can become so immersed in their roles that they no longer recognise how they truly feel about *anything*. They are so lost in their new, assumed identity that they get totally disconnected from their true feelings.

Each role, assumed for acceptance, is characterised by different behaviour patterns, but they all share one thing in common: they represent the loss of connection to the authentic self. If you feel that you are playing a role, you can decide if it serves you or if you would like to shift into what is perhaps a more authentic version of yourself. If we want to free ourselves from contrived role-playing, there are things we can address, for example:

*The '**Super-Achiever/Hero**' can learn that it's OK to be a human being rather than a 'human do-ing'. It's OK to not be perfect and it's OK to ask for help and be vulnerable.

> ## Releasing My Roles
> *While I was obese, I was a definite 'people-pleaser', along with 'super-achiever' and probably most of the other roles mentioned here. I had little self-confidence and was embroiled in over-busyness, looking for acceptance anywhere I thought I might get it. When I started my transformation, I found it really hard to give up these old roles and patterns. My boundaries were very 'flimsy' and I'd agree to help with almost any task, scattering my energy in multiple directions. Through exploring various 'self-help' tools – such as those in the Guidance section of this book – I gradually learned to relax and get my boundaries more into line. I came to recognise my own true needs and desires, to say 'NO' when it felt healthy, to stop participating in shaming/sarcastic interactions and so on. There were many awkward feelings for me to work through. For so long I'd blocked so much out, kept so much down, never felt the feelings, never shared honestly. It was a time of massive release for me and I was so grateful to emerge into the 'light' on the other side as a more authentic, joyful version of my self.*

*The '**People-Pleaser/Nice Guy**' can learn that it's OK to say no if they want to, that it's OK to say what they really think/feel and that other people can do things for themselves.

*The '**Scapegoat**' can learn that it's OK to reveal any hurt feelings underneath the rage, it's OK to stop rebelling and start negotiating, to say no without being hostile and to seek support.

*The '**Lost Child**' can learn that it's OK to reach out to others, to face issues instead of disappearing into hobbies; it's OK to be seen by others for who we really are and to have close relationships.

*The '**Mascot/Joker**' can learn that it's OK to assume responsibility, to let others entertain themselves, and to 'risk' being serious or assertive.

We may find that we identify with aspects of several roles, as we are seldom strictly confined to one, assuming different roles depending on the situation. Whichever pattern(s) we may associate with, the important message to understand is that we can take steps to move out of our assumed roles, if we want to embody a more authentic version of ourselves. Many of the tools and tips shared below in the Guidance section will help you to tune into your 'real' self and drop the mask.

Boundary / Trust Issues

One of the keys for solid recovery is defining our boundaries - what is and isn't acceptable for us in communication with others. The boundaries we set for ourselves define who we are and how we allow others to treat us. Boundaries are often a big issue for healing, as few of us grew up with very healthy role models of communication. Areas to address typically include standing by what we believe in (even if others feel differently), learning to get our needs met healthily and practicing saying no. Saying no when you don't want to participate in something is vital for creating healthy boundaries and only you can know when 'no'

The Girl Who Forgot How to Say 'No'

*As an infant, my very first word was 'no', so it seems reasonable to assume that I'd have had enough practice with this word over the years to freely use it as required. Yet, this wasn't really the case. As a morbidly obese young woman, my boundaries seemed almost limitless towards others. I felt like I 'just couldn't say no'. I'd agree to participate in anything and everything that I thought might bring me attention, acceptance or **approval**. The number of groups and volunteering organisations I participated in at University, for example, at the height of my obesity, was extraordinary. I was writing for this newspaper, serving on the board of that committee, starting this society, radio producing here, singing there, learning sign language, helping in a day centre for head injuries, out in the woods doing conservation work and so on – all while studying full time. As a side benefit, I enjoyed giving the impression of being 'far too busy' for that which I really could have benefited from: honesty, love and a genuine connection with my true self and others. Though I wasn't truly happy, this 'protection bubble' I'd created for myself at least felt secure and I didn't want to disturb that...*
I almost always agreed with anything people said and put their needs before mine, rather than using that simple little word – 'no' – and facing the possibility that someone might disagree with me. I lived in constant fear of rejection and disapproval. These days, thankfully, things are very different. My boundaries are far clearer, as I get into better contact with who I really am and what I want and need. If I don't want to do something now, or don't agree with something, I feel free to say 'no', without fear of abandonment. It is OK for me to be who I am, to have my needs and feelings and it is definitely OK for me to connect again to that infant me and say 'no'.

is right for you. When you first start saying no, you might feel guilty - be aware that this is a common experience and don't let it stop you doing what feels true for you. It is important to put your *own* needs first. You cannot have healthy relationships with others without good boundaries, so remember that laying down limits is a loving thing to do. Seek healthy communication with people who respect your boundaries and don't attempt to tell you what you 'should' be doing. Above all, seek to get what you need emotionally in healthy *relationships*, rather than from eating.

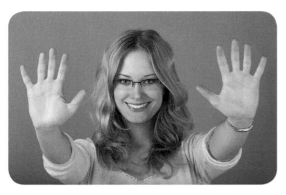

It is not uncommon to have trust issues alongside boundary issues, usually stemming from an early decision that the world around us is not a safe place to express our true selves. Through seeking out 'safe' people who are physically, emotionally and spiritually available, we can begin to build trust and genuine intimacy with others.

Co-dependency

Co dependency is another common trait that can be defined as an urgent desire for affirmation from others, without which one may feel lost, unwanted and unlovable. This is learned behaviour. We also learn to put the opinions and feelings of others before our own needs and feelings when our self-worth is not valued. Eminent self-help writer Charles L. Whitfield defines co-dependency as: 'Suffering and dysfunction associated with or due to focusing on the needs or behaviours of others'.

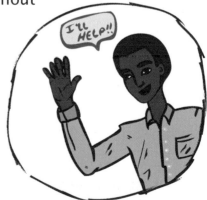

Co-dependent behaviours may include:

*Difficulty making decisions
*Judging oneself as not good enough
*Embarrassed by recognition/praise/gifts
*Compliance: compromising values/integrity to avoid rejection/anger

*Basing one's own feelings on how others seem to feel
*Getting resentful if others don't want to be helped
*Offering advice without being asked
*Lavishing gifts and favours on others

Co-dependents have learned to look to others for acknowledgement that they are acceptable. They also typically display low self-esteem and preoccupation with the opinions and behaviour of others, ignore their own feelings, blame themselves if things go 'wrong', over-extend themselves into other peoples' lives and stay in situations that are damaging to them out of 'loyalty'. Co-dependents frequently either exaggerate things or grossly underplay them with self-deprecating statements like 'I'm terrible at this' or 'I'm the worst person at doing this in the world'. These can all be subversive ways of trying to find affirmation and attention.

If this all sounds familiar, the Guidance section below is going to be a great aid for you. You might also find it useful to read a book such as *Co-dependent No More* by Melody Beattie or attend 'Co-dependents Anonymous' meetings to help release unsupportive patterns (see the Resources section for more information).

Shame

In our modern societies, it seems that many of us experience shaming as children and little acceptance of our true selves. There's a big difference between 'healthy' and 'toxic' shame. 'Healthy' shame is a common human feeling that tells us something about our limits. For example, sometimes we are not able to do everything we want to do by ourselves; we could use some help, we may blush, feel shy and so on. Unhealthy or 'toxic' shame, on the other hand, is like an all-pervasive sense of being flawed, far beyond any fleeting sense of inadequacy. People living with toxic shame usually feel worthless and defective.

Toxic shame can develop for numerous reasons. When we do not receive adequate mirroring from our caregivers as children, or in our adult relationships, we're not seen or affirmed for who we really are; rather we are moulded and conditioned to fit others' expectations. We may frequently be told 'no' and any legitimate feelings such as anger may be denied or repressed; we are blamed and shamed for doing things that are actually perfectly natural stages of development (e.g. picking things up and putting them in our mouth as toddlers). We may thereby come to believe that we are not acceptable as we are and thus must be flawed. As the shame transforms into a toxic identity, we block out our real feelings and needs and often turn to an addiction (e.g. overeating) to numb the pain. We live with low self-worth and a sense of being inherently flawed, searching for happiness, success or fulfilment in all kinds of places, other than within ourselves. Food addicts tend to search in the fridge, but that is not where true peace and happiness are to be found. No matter how much chocolate or cake we eat, it is never enough to fill the gaping black chasm of emotional and spiritual emptiness within.

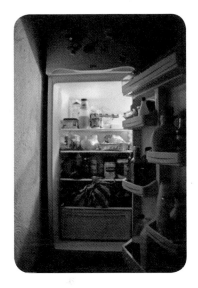

This process of toxic shame is frequently acknowledged as the core of most forms of emotional illness, including compulsive disorders, depression, perfectionism, paranoia, inferiority complexes and alienation. Be particularly on the watch for sarcasm – this is a common form of shaming that is passed off as humour.

Defences

We may use defences to protect our addiction/false identity and keep feelings at bay so that (for food addicts) we feel we can justify ourselves and continue overeating. Typical defences include:

Denial - 'I can stop whenever I want'.
Minimising - 'It's not that much of an issue'.
Rationalising - 'I could be knocked down by a bus anyway'.
Entitlement - 'I deserve this, I've worked hard today'.
Blame - 'If I didn't have to put up with this/him/her, I'd stop'.
Self-pity - 'I'm so busy/overwhelmed/weak. It's too hard to stop'.

Worrying about things instead of being present in the moment is another form of defence. Worry doesn't prevent disaster, it prevents joy. Becoming aware of which defences you use and how you use them is another valuable step towards being able to make choices about your behaviour in the future. By recognising your defence patterns rather than ignoring them, you can choose to set them aside. If you then decide to keep using your defences, however, it will at least be a conscious choice rather than a reflex response.

Control Issues

Many of us develop control issues as coping mechanisms in childhood, after receiving (often indirect) messages such as 'always stay in control' and 'if things don't go as planned, find someone to blame'. In our current lives, these control patterns may show up as having set thoughts about how things/people 'should' be, making resentful judgements about anything that doesn't fit our personal model and so on. Our frustration at things not working out exactly as we want may manifest in various ways: silent aggression, outright rage, isolation/withdrawal, violence, manipulation and so on. However, these outdated coping mechanisms really serve no-one. As much as we may want to, we cannot make anyone else's choices for them and control *everything*. The only things we really have total choice about are *our* own attitudes and behaviour.

Perfectionism

Many of us make perfectionistic demands on ourselves and others, based on our model of what we consider to be 'right'. This is another coping mechanism developed to survive unhealthy environments where we may have received messages from parent figures such as 'always do the right thing' and 'it's unforgivable to make mistakes'. A perfectionist might think and

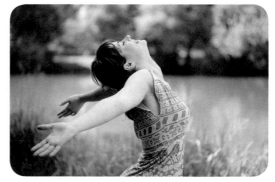

speak in terms of things they 'have' to do, 'should' do, 'must do' and so on. You do not ever *have* to do anything; you are free to make choices in every moment.

Now, as adults, we can more easily reflect and accept for ourselves that we are fallible, that we sometimes do things in a way that seems other than optimal and it's all perfectly OK. We do not have to be perfect and we do not have to accept shaming, blaming or criticism from anyone, ourselves included, when we do make what are perceived as errors. We also do not have to live with regret and remorse about anything we judge as 'imperfect' about our past.

Next time you're 'putting yourself down', consider this: would you speak to a friend in the way you are addressing yourself? We can be so harsh on ourselves. Relax and show yourself some self-love. Rather than focusing on what you consider 'wrong' or 'imperfect' about yourself, take note of the things you appreciate and enjoy. What did you do today that was fun, uplifting, creative, served somebody else? Try focusing your energy towards these positive elements of your behaviour instead and more will surely follow. Learning to accept compliments without minimising or ignoring the praise, or resorting to self-criticism/sarcasm, is another useful skill for healing.

'Unhealthy' Relationships

When we start out on our path of healing, many of us are involved in de-energised, toxic and conflict-ridden relationships. Intimacy and genuine enjoyment with others may have become overshadowed by our eating. We might have isolated ourselves in our relationship with food, seeking only instant intimacy from what we eat and ignoring everything else. Now, as we step into active transformation, it can be very nourishing for all involved if we address 'unhealthy' relationship issues and move towards intimacy with others that includes safe sharing of feelings.

Examining or even letting go of unhealthy relationships that no longer serve us can feel **very** challenging. However, take an honest look at the relationships you share with those around you. How do you feel when you interact with these people? Do you feel love, support, encouragement, acceptance? Or do you feel drained, weakened, judged or even *ridiculed*? Do others treat you as you treat them?

When we start to make positive, uplifting shifts in our lives, the people around us may not want to come along with us on that path. For example, in some families where most people are heavy, it might perversely seem like 'going against the rules' to even lose weight and get healthy. Be vigilant of your boundaries at this time – remember that you are free to choose your own path at every

Hello! Hello…???

It's been interesting for me to see the reactions of old friends since I went raw, lost weight and experienced such a dramatic transformation. Most seemed shocked. Having lived in many different places with many different people, I have friends scattered all over the world. Most didn't know about my transformation as it unfolded. Months or years later I would meet up with people and they literally wouldn't recognise me. I found it rather entertaining!

I recall meeting one friend at Piccadilly Circus in London. She was there before me and I saw her as I approached. I walked nearer…and nearer…and nearer…until I was about four feet away from her. She was blanking me: she couldn't see me, even though I was right there in front of her, because the physical form I now embodied didn't match the image in her memory. She saw the form of a woman moving closer to her and thought it was someone coming to 'bother' her. The last time we'd met, I was around 300 pounds – now I was around 145. More than half of me was gone and she didn't recognise me. She even looked me in the face a couple of times, before suddenly it all clicked and she realised it was me. She was very surprised and we laughed a great deal as we reconnected and I told her all about my new raw lifestyle.

*I like this story, because I feel it relates through **physical** form an experience many of us seem to have when we reconnect with old friends who don't seem willing/able to see the 'new' us that has emerged in the time we've been apart. In this instance, my friend couldn't see me standing right there in front of her, because the body form I was now in didn't match her memory.*

*How many of us have experienced big transformations in our lives, then felt as if we're 'not seen' when we meet again with people who knew us before? There's a strong tendency to slip back into old roles/patterns in such instances, so that everyone feels 'comfortable'. In contrast, my dramatic change in **physical form** (aside from the other shifts I'd experienced on all levels) seemed hard for many people from my past to really integrate, as it was such a visible, 'in-your-face' change, which wasn't going away. It couldn't be glossed over and easily ignored.*

I'm really not the same person anymore, I don't fit the pattern of what used to be 'Angela' and this newness seemed peculiar and even perhaps 'threatening' in some way to the reality of some older friends. I recall one person for example feeling unable to look me in the eye when we first met again after I'd lost all the weight – it was extraordinary to witness. It seemed to me as if she literally couldn't 'face' the shifts. People tend to like things to feel comfortably familiar and to stay the same… My metamorphosis was pretty extreme and seemed to jar the comfort zones of many people around me…

As mentioned elsewhere, these days the vast majority of my social interactions are with other raw foodies, who seem to readily embrace the 'new me'. For this I am grateful.

moment. If someone dear to you is unwilling to support your journey, it might be kindest (for all involved) to minimise or even suspend contact for a while. Things may shift again in the future and your paths may **reconnect**. For the time being though, if your relationship no longer feels supportive, it would be very wise to look for community with others who do understand your path. You cannot make anyone else's choices for them, so it seems much simpler to seek out those who are like-minded rather than trying to 'make' things that matter greatly to you fit into a relationship that feels strained. This is not to suggest that we all ought to up and leave our current communities when we start to heal. In fact, I truly believe that it is possible to live together and hold loving space with *anyone*, if you choose to do it. Indeed, the impact of one person making positive shifts can ripple out through a whole community in amazing ways. Nonetheless, it is true that interacting with *some* people is going to feel like much more of an energy-drain than a boost. Therefore I recommend fostering connections with those who already understand and support your experiences, as one way of simplifying and lightening the load.

Choose to be around those in whose presence you feel energetic, creative and uplifted. Be wary, in particular, of 'toxic' individuals who manipulate, rage and throw tantrums regularly (rather than occasionally) and without remorse. It is likely the kindest move for all involved if you cease attempting to get love and support from a person whose behaviour seems toxic in this way. Seeking support from people like this can be compared to going to a clothes boutique to try to buy peaches; you're not looking in an appropriate place. Instead, follow your highest truth, pray for the other person and send him or her a lot of **love and healing**.

If a romantic relationship in your life ends, be honest about why it ended and - if you feel like it's useful – seek constructive feedback from others about their perspective on this matter. This can help us to gain clarity about what we don't want to repeat/choose next time. We can then focus more clearly on what we *are* reaching for – rather than what we are leaving behind. We can nurture our self-worth and inner beloved, then start moving towards a healthy relationship with someone who seems like a more appropriate match for this stage in our journey.

Now that we've taken a good look at the different kinds of patterns, thought processes, addictions, issues and more that can bubble up for release during emotional detox, let's move on to taking ACTION. We know now what we're dealing with, so, what are we going to do about it? It's time to delve into the Guidance section and explore tips, ideas and activities for your glowing, active transformation...

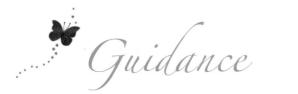

Guidance

Time to Fill *Your* Treasure Box -
Your Companion for Maintenance

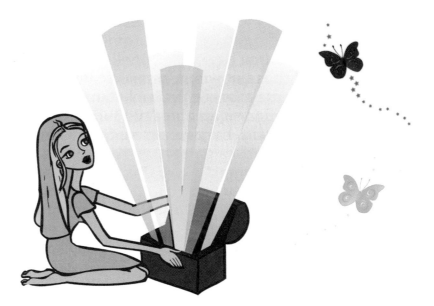

When we're lost in cycles of using food compulsively, it can seem like *eating* is essential for us to feel good. Yet in truth, so much more joy, exhilaration, fun and deep satisfaction can be experienced if we step away from the food and get more actively engaged in other aspects of life. You can start to *really* enjoy yourself and have healthy, satisfying fun without guilt, remorse or extra pounds. Think of all the other exciting things you could be engaging your emotions with beyond food – exercise, gatherings with friends, reading, dancing, learning new skills and so on. These are the kind of alternatives we'll be exploring in this section. You will find sixty different inspirational ideas for transformation, intended to help you release old patterns, divided into twenty Recovery Concepts and forty Healthy Action Tips. You can consider this collection your 'Treasure Box' of guidance to help smooth your journey from the Realisation/Transition stages to a happy, healthy life of Maintenance.

The tools and guidance we can access to help us along this journey are myriad. The paths are many, the truth is one. In the end, it really makes no difference which tools/techniques you use as long as you feel good about them – this is the most important thing. One person, for example, may find Reiki outstanding for their emotional well-being, while someone else barely notices its effect. We all have different preferences and responses. There is no 'magic answer' that fits everyone – it is about aligning with what raises your *own* vibration. Play with whatever genuinely connects, holds and inspires *you*, remembering that while healing can sometimes feel like work, often the greatest healing involves *fun*.

I'm going to share here some of the tools that I recommend and which have been the most useful for *me* in my recovery. All of these can be used in preference to focusing on food or overeating as a way to help shift your mood and emotions, although this is by no means an exhaustive list.

Remember that the suggestions here represent a *selection* of healing tools available to us. It may be that none of them 'fit' you exactly. That's OK – look for something else that does or mix a few different techniques. Also remember that none of these tools represent 'the' answer for your fulfilment and feeling of connection. The true source for happiness is always *within* – choose not to focus your energy *outwards* to some object, technique or person as if they are the source of your health, happiness and well-being. Such outer resources are simply islands of inspiration, guidance and support on your way. Just as *food* is not 'the answer' for true happiness, neither are the suggestions given below – try not to simply transfer any sense of addiction.

If we also choose to see this whole transformation process as one of using tools to discard old behaviours that do not serve us well, rather than 'a battle to overcome our desires', this can be a joyful and rewarding experience.

The twenty **Recovery Concepts** are guiding principles that you might find useful to examine and apply in your life. You may feel moved to start incorporating them *all* at once, or you might find it more manageable to work with one or more at a time, gently integrating them into your new awareness and patterns.

The forty Healthy Action Tips are much more focused on *activities*. If you tried to incorporate all of these in one go, I think it would almost certainly feel overwhelming! Therefore, to begin with, I suggest picking three of the suggestions here that most appeal to you and trying them out. See where this takes you. You can choose more to experiment with later.

Take your time to adjust to these new lifestyle suggestions, rather than stressing yourself into overwhelm about ALL the new things you may want to experience. You do not have to do everything at once to start seeing and feeling a positive difference in your life. Remember that recovery is an ongoing process, not a one-off event. This '**Treasure Box**' of suggestions is yours to open up and dip into whenever you like – it is always here for you.

All the tips shared here can be used as both day-to-day ongoing preventative 'remedies' for relieving self-destructive patterns and as 'band-aids' in times of craving crises. Just open this book, delve into your Treasure Box and find something to inspire you, beyond the food! If you are diligent and consistently engage some of these suggestions in your daily life, you will naturally find yourself experiencing fewer cravings anyway, as your energy will be regularly directed elsewhere (i.e., other than towards eating).

When you *do* try something out, I encourage you to give it a 'fair go', rather than trying it for perhaps half an hour and then dismissing it. New behaviours and ideas may seem to fit awkwardly into our landscape at first – you can think of this like 'breaking in' a new pair of shoes. Persistence pays off: the edges will soften and you might find yourself with a vastly more comfortable and enjoyable outlook. You might also enjoy writing a short-list for yourself of all the suggestions below that really resonate for you – the activities and non-food treats you LOVE – then post this list up on your fridge door. Next time you find yourself reaching towards the fridge, you'll see that the 'answer' is ON the fridge, rather than IN it...!

Twenty Core Recovery Concepts

We start with twenty basic recovery concepts to help shape your transformation. These are presented here in no particular order. You can use them as touchstones to refer back to throughout your healing, to see how your perspective is shifting.

Look Within

One of the greatest gifts I've been given in my life was when a dear elder friend told me, 'You have everything you need within yourself. You do not need to look anywhere else for answers.' This was a turning point in my life and it can be for you too, if you are willing to open to the universal truth: that we all have access to all the answers we are looking for, right inside ourselves. Give up assuming that the answers you search for are outside yourself. You do not need any 'guru' to lead the way – you are connected to all that you need, right now. We all have available the same access, the same connection to the Divine. It may take a little effort for you to become quiet enough to hear and listen to that still, small voice within, yet do not doubt that it is there – it is within us all. Learn to trust your own intuition; your feelings are your guide.

Everybody wants to feel happy. Many of us tell ourselves stories that things will be 'perfect' in life *once* we have the right body shape/partner/dress size and so on. We often seem to believe that happiness will come from an external source. When we get into emotional recovery, we learn that happiness is ours to have at any time and that it comes from within. If we invest our sense of happiness in other people/things, then we give our power away and become dependent on them to feel happy. We do not have to live in pain, boredom and frustration, waiting for some point of perfection in a distant and imaginary future. All we have is *now*, and misery – just like happiness – is a choice.

> *"It is not easy to find happiness in ourselves*
> *and it is not possible to find it elsewhere."*
> *--Agnes Repplier*

Go For It – and Follow Through

New experiences and exercises with 'self-development' work can sometimes feel a bit odd and tricky. You may feel embarrassed and self-conscious, yet transcend this and it will definitely be worthwhile. *Commit* to investing time and energy in your transformation and remind yourself that you are worth it. Taking shortcuts in recovery doesn't pay. If you find yourself minimising

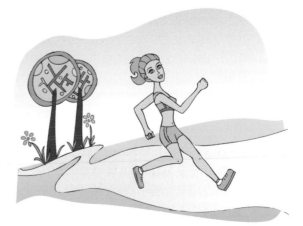

the time you devote to self-development, consider how much time you used to spend eating excess amounts, thinking of food, visiting shops and restaurants and apply all that time instead to doing your active transformation work (and play). Accept that everything you do and everything you put your attention towards is simply a choice. Stop making 'excuses' for yourself if you do not do something that you had intended to do. There is no need for justification, excuses or reasoning – it all comes down to your choice.

Imagine, for example, that you would like to be doing an hour of exercise daily, yet never seem to do that. You get the same amount of hours in a day as everybody else, yet one person might consistently do ninety minutes of exercise a day, while you find you actually manage ten minutes, three times a week. You can come up with any number of reasons, justifications and excuses as to why – ultimately, it is really neither here nor there. The time is as available to exercise for you as it is for anyone else; it is simply a matter of where you are choosing to put your attention. Quit spinning your wheels in excuses! If you really want to do something, try committing to what you say you want to do and following through. If it doesn't happen, that's OK, it just means that you put your attention somewhere else in the end. It is always a simple matter of choice, nothing more, nothing less and *your* choice is *your* responsibility.

A Bonus Boundary Tip
We've already taken a look at boundaries - honouring your own wants and needs in response to others. Keep on strengthening your boundaries and take note of this extra tip:

Once you feel that you've established healthy boundaries, learn to protect them, to take care of yourself. A helpful way to do this is to imagine a flexible fence all around you, with which you can let people as near to you as you find comfortable, depending on how 'safe' you feel with them. If someone seems very honest, open, non-judgemental and supportive, you can choose to swing a gate gently open to them, allowing them closer. If, however, you experience someone as shaming, blaming or judging you, you may want to expand the perimeter of your fence, with bolts securely in place around you, to make your position vibrationally clear. You can emanate love, support and compassion towards that person, just do so from a place where you feel safe.

166

Simplify

How clear does your living space look? It is common in our modern societies to lead hectic, stressful lives in houses that are cluttered with *things*, which many times bring us little to no real joy. We are immersed in distractions. Our cities epitomise a culture focused on anything but self-reflection and connection. People travel to work at jobs they don't enjoy to make money to spend on things and activities that bring minimal genuine satisfaction. Indeed, modern city life often seems like a perverse competition of who can be the most strung-out and stressed. People try to keep up with all the news and events going on around them and exhaust themselves through involvement with so much information and technology.

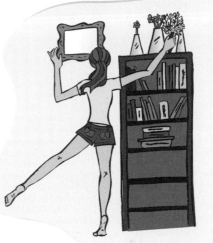

Take a look at your own life and patterns. How much time do you take in a day to check in with yourself about how you really feel? How connected to your true self do you actually feel? How many hours do you take instead for activities which, in honesty, bring you no deep satisfaction? How much time do you devote to focusing on how *other* people seem to feel – those you read about in magazines, watch on TV or listen to on the radio? Watch out for these things that distract you from an intrinsic connection with your self and thus the whole. Weed these 'clutter activities' out of your life – in short, *simplify*.

Turn off your TV and computer for a while, unplug your phone – take some valuable 'me' time instead. Limiting your exposure to mainstream media can help enormously to get on track with your own desires, away from all those advertisements, product placements, depressing stories and pressures to conform.

It is much easier to live a focused, raw, positive 'alternative' lifestyle when you are not giving attention to that mainstream model of reality. Recognise the illusion of fast-paced city life for what it is and the fact that it is not necessary to live in that way, so out of touch with nature. Nature is about simplicity. Remove objects from your home that no longer serve or bring you delight, cancel activities from your schedule that keep you distracted and stressed, enjoy time in nature, practice regular meditation and…relax… ;)

"What is this life if, full of care,
We have no time to stand and stare?"
--W.H. Davies

Live, Love, Let Go

When times feel tough, use some of the tools outlined here, breathe deeply and *let go.* Staying attached to outcomes or viewing situations as a 'problem' (as opposed to an opportunity) will never serve you. Don't try to push things to fit your expectations – instead, learn to accept what you cannot change (especially other people's behaviour) and allow things to flow. There can be a tendency for people to get locked in to their own perspective and inflexibly believe it to be 'the right way'. If things are not panning out as *you* would like, take an energetic side-step and focus your attention elsewhere for a while. There is always something else positive to focus upon.

Surrendering does not mean giving up, it means letting go of the outcome. Be flexible, open and adaptable.

Be aware that 'what you resist, persists' – if you don't appreciate someone else's behaviour in a situation and you resist it, rather than letting go and creating a space of love between the two of you, the irritation can easily persist.

Learn to accept that nothing is personal; we are all connected and reflect different aspects of each other. Often, if you notice something in someone else that irritates you – e.g. you find them arrogant – it is simply because you have not yet fully accepted, integrated and forgiven that part of *yourself.* In this way, they reflect that aspect of your being back at you, like a mirror. You can use clues like this to assist your own healing, if you are willing.

If you can view your experiences here on Earth as a game, with yourself as the observer, watching for clues and following leads, it is much easier to let go. See uncomfortable situations as 'stormy weather' moving through your landscape. Know that this too shall pass. Have faith that you will be carried. Look at every challenge as an opportunity. We are all here to experience, co-create and enjoy and holding on to 'sticky' emotions certainly complicates this. As the saying goes:

> *"All that really matters in the end,*
> *Is how much did you **live**,*
> *How much did you love,*
> *How much did you learn to let go...?"*

The Only Constant Is Change

Things in life continuously flow and shift. You may find yourself clinging to the idea that at some point you're going to reach a 'perfect' place with your food or body or *anything* and that from then on, all will be excellent. It seldom works this way. Life is an endless dance of interacting energies and just as soon as it might seem like things have drawn to a stop, another thread will be rising up to intertwine in the endless and often beautiful web we weave together. This process never ends. We might have a 'to do' list, scratch out the last item on it and gain some divine moments of blissful 'completion', then it's in with the new and on with the show... For

Get On With It

During my own transformation, I saw how resistant I can be to change – even very positive shifts. I'd create blocks against starting things, pushing things to one side 'for later' and various other procrastination techniques. I was always waiting for the 'perfect' moment to do something, yet more often than not, that perfect moment would never arrive. The things I resisted could involve anything, from trying a new recipe to writing an important letter to quitting a job. Slowly, after simply acknowledging this behaviour, I was able to gently bring myself to try out and enjoy new things much faster, rather than procrastinating.

It takes courage to change, yet usually I find that I feel really happy and inspired after making even simple changes. Just taking baby steps, like picking up and reading a few pages of an inspiring book, can feel hugely beneficial. Once I allow myself to make a change and come out glowing on the other side, I often wonder why it took me so long to do it in the first place. I find it helps to remind myself that shifts don't have to be scary and don't have to involve permanent alterations. I can simply try things out and the more I let go and become open to new experiences, the easier and more enjoyable I find life to be.

There is not and never will be a 'perfect' time to do anything, other than right now. This moment is all we have and this moment is a precious opportunity. If you are given the inspiration to try something, follow the lead - it may result in some wonderful unfoldings for you. The key thing is really to enjoy all that you choose to experience. We have the choice in this and every moment to feel joy.

me, this felt like a particularly tricky aspect of life to integrate. I didn't *want* it all to keep shifting all the time. I wanted it to stop and be 'easy', not constantly a-flow with new input: emails, trips, meetings, planning, events and so on...and yet, in truth, a life *devoid* of flow and spontaneity would never really keep me joyful on this journey.

How many people do you know who settle into a 'comfortable' life of mediocrity that brings them no true sense of satisfaction? Well, stagnating over pre-packaged TV meals in suburbia is never quite going to do it for me. So it is that I seek to embrace change and accept the joy of standing up strong and riding the wave of transformation as it works its way through my life, rather than sitting meekly on the shoreline. I prefer the path of the passionate transformer – invite *yourself* to share that path too!

Compassion

Try making a habit of seeing the divinity and light in everyone you encounter, from shop assistants to police officers to farmers to people living on the streets. If ever you sense reservation, imagine your heart opening in acceptance of this other being. Let others know that you appreciate who they are/what they do and *why*, remembering that everyone is doing their best in every given moment. (For example, you might let the gardeners in your local park know that you appreciate the work they do there *because* it brings you such pleasure to see the beautiful flowers and trees.) *You* have the power of love within you in any given moment to help brighten the lives of others. Practice seeing everyone as your brothers and sisters and know that, if even one amongst us feels uncomfortable, this affects the whole. We are all connected and our every thought and action ripples out beyond us.

Personally, since going raw, I've been amazed how my sense of compassion and love for others has expanded. In my past, I was very insular and felt easily irritated by others. In contrast, it's common these days for me to sit in a bus full of people and feel such beautiful, silent waves of love for everyone there. It feels so much more comfortable to me to sense and honour the divinity in everyone like that, than to be quietly criticising all around me instead, in my head.

If you find someone's behaviour irritating, try pulling away the masks of 'appearance' and imagining them as a five-year-old child, lost and looking for love and attention in whatever way they can, wounded and vulnerable. (Or even more effec-

170

tive: try to see them as a five-year-old version of *yourself* – wouldn't you like that little person to be handled with love, compassion and understanding?) As we've already considered, often what we find irritating in others is as much about the same quality in *ourselves* that, for some reason, we do not lovingly accept. Forgiveness is always two-fold and is primarily a gift to oneself. It is an all-round wonderful gift when you spread kindness and generosity, help uplift others and genuinely listen. At first it may feel scary and even 'burdensome' to be the one giving love towards others, especially if it seems they are not reciprocating. Yet know this: all that you give out comes back to you manifold and attracts even more joy, compassion and prosperity for all.

Being able to feel compassion for others begins with accepting and forgiving *ourselves*. It takes courage to uncover the pain we may be holding within and embrace all our feelings with compassion, yet it is a key practice for transformation.

Find Your Bliss

Get clear about what you really want in life. Many people are unclear about what it is they're doing here. If you don't clearly define what you'd like to see and experience, you are unlikely to be following a path that brings you real fulfillment and joy. Choose work that you love. Do what you love and love what you do. What is it that you're best at? What most holds your attention and brings you joy? What would you do with your time if you were *guaranteed* to feel successful and fulfilled with it? When we follow the true path of our heart's desire, unimaginable things can unfold. Once we get clear about what it is we really want to focus our energy towards, the Universe rushes in to support us. We no longer sit watching clocks and waiting for vacations; we LOVE our *vocations* instead.

As we honour our choices and follow our bliss, we feel amazingly empowered and our self-trust also rebuilds. This is an area where women in particular tend to feel confused and disconnected. Many women are so accustomed to giving their power and energy away to others that they are unclear what they really want or enjoy for *themselves*. Take a while to examine your life – get honest – what brings you the most joy? Which activities do you start doing and find hours pass without you even noticing? These are clues and the answers will be different for everyone. For one person it might be fixing up motorbikes, while another loves patchwork quilts. Ultimately, it really doesn't matter what it is, as long as you align with what *you* love to do. The real concern is that you *love* what you are putting your attention towards. Get out of your head and into your heart. What does *your* heart desire?

"Well-behaved women rarely make history."
--Laurel Thatcher Ulrich

STOP and THINK

When the compulsion to overeat or to consume Trigger foods comes to you, stop and ask yourself, 'What is it that I'm trying to not feel?' Remember that overeating is a *coping* mechanism we have been using to block our real feelings. Before you reach for the cookie tin, **stop** and **think**: '*where* is this craving coming from?' When you realise what you've been trying to avoid – for example, feeling nervous about an upcoming interview – then you can acknowledge that you feel afraid, perhaps by speaking it out loud to a loved one, or writing it down, then channel your energy elsewhere. This is a very simple and effective strategy for acknowledging and embracing your feelings, dissipating the energy and allowing it to pass. Whatever you do, try not to hold onto your feelings, deny them or block their passing. Ask Spirit for help, speak to someone else, write, send an email or whatever it takes; just don't keep things locked up inside.

Avoiding Assumptions

It can be very easy to get our 'wires crossed' with others when we live by assumptions. If you find yourself, for example, with hands on hips saying to a loved one, 'You KNOW I didn't want to come here' or perhaps watching *their* face fall as you tell them, 'I didn't get you a ticket, because I knew you wouldn't enjoy it', it might be time to reassess how clearly you communicate. Making *assumptions* about another person's perspective is rarely the most direct route to understanding their desires. Asserting also that they 'must' surely know what you would like/want/dislike and so on is an equally unclear way to communicate. Be clear in stating your own feelings/desires and asking others about theirs. If you pay attention to each person's actual *truth* more and assume less, you'll very likely find that your communications improve and your misunderstandings dwindle.

LISTEN

It is shocking to me how many people seem to feel that they do not have someone in their life who *truly* listens to them. Everyone wants to be heard and acknowledged for their perspective. Yet it seems that, in conversation, people are often more focused on having their *own* voices heard than on listening to anyone else. Remember to treat everyone as you would have yourself treated: 'do as you would be done by'. If you want to genuinely be heard, begin by genuinely listening to others. Refrain from interrupting others, speaking over them or using body language, e.g. yawns, coughs and so on, to interrupt their flow. If you find yourself doing any of these, use this awareness to return your focus to listening. As you listen, notice and switch off any inner impulse to formulate your response – simply listen to the speaker and what they want to share. Remember too that when you talk, you usually just repeat what *you* already know; when you *listen* (or read) instead, you often learn something new.

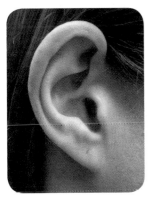

Slow down, maintain eye contact with whomever you're listening to, give affirmative nods, gestures or sounds if this feels appropriate and let them share. Many of us were not brought up to feel secure about the validity of our perspective. As children we may have been frequently talked over, dismissed or told that we were 'wrong' without being given a reason why. Do your best now to help others feel confident as they speak – their opinion and desire to express is just as valid as anyone else's.

A simple way to affirm this to someone is to tell them 'I hear you' when they have finished speaking. Once you have heard them out, you might reaffirm this by paraphrasing some of what has been said and sharing what this means to you. Pay attention to any feedback they might then give you on your reflections; remain open to refreshing your perspective accordingly.

In my work as a raw lifestyle consultant, it is clear to me that many people are simply looking for an outlet to speak about their issues without judgement, criticism or shame. People are looking for a safe context in which to express themselves. Try your best to be a beacon of healing communication in *your* community and hold the space for others to express. Be an active transformer. As you do so, others will reciprocate and your relationship dynamics may shift dramatically.

Take Responsibility

If you are prone to telling stories about what others have 'done to you' to enable yourself to blame others for your situation and stay in a victim role, learn to recognise this behaviour and leave it behind. The situation you find

> ## Taking Responsibility for *My* Food Choices
>
> *Bread was the most difficult thing for me to 'give up' when I went raw. I was deeply addicted to wheat and would often eat bread products three (or more) times a day: toast with breakfast, sandwiches at lunch, bread and butter as a side dish with dinner... I recall clearly my attempts to manipulate my partner of the time while I was transitioning away from bread. I tried to transfer some of the responsibility for what I ate onto him, by creating 'rules' like: 'If you see me eat more than three pieces of bread with this meal, please stop me'. I clearly see now how I was attempting to offset my choices and responsibility for my food intake onto him. I didn't want to be the one 'policing' my own bread intake, so I tried to get him to take on that role instead. I laugh now when I think of this story, as I cannot imagine asking somebody to perform such a role anymore. I guess addictions can really foster some odd behaviour... I'm also happy to say that in the end I took responsibility for my **own** choices and omitted the bread. These days romaine wraps, flax crackers, raw pizza bases and so on more than satisfy me. Now I can't imagine even wanting to eat sliced white bread...*

yourself in is a result of your *own* choices. Not taking responsibility for yourself in this way creates a big obstacle to recovery. Recognise that things happen **through you**, rather than **to** you. You are one of countless conduits for the universal energy and you are co-creating in every moment with *your* free-will choices.

A very common way that people use blaming language in our cultures is with statements like 'you *make* me feel sad', 'she *made* me feel so small' and so on. Nobody can **make** you feel or do anything – it is all a choice, in every single moment. Move away from such disempowering language; step up and take responsibility for what you are feeling and where you are directing your energy. As an example, if you feel upset because someone didn't meet you when they said they would, instead of saying to them 'you made me upset', try something like 'When you didn't come at the agreed time, I felt sad. I really wanted to connect with you.' **Remove the blame** and claim your own feelings.

Separation is just an illusion; we are all connected, so try to treat *everything* you encounter as 'sacred' and a part of you. Maybe somebody else dropped that piece of litter near you, for example – you could still pick it up. It's your environment to enjoy too; we are all guardians here. Exchange blaming and finger-pointing for *being the change* – remember, you're an 'active transformer'. Make your own impact in the world match your vision of what you most love to see and experience. Take responsibility for being a beacon for the positive changes you desire and this can inspire others to step up too.

If you are experiencing issues in a relationship and *you* are conscious of that, try taking responsibility for your part in healing any disharmony. Step away from the victim role and acknowledge that you have co-created the situation together. Rather than trying to blame your parents/doctor/psychiatrist/partner for a situation, assume responsibility for your part in that co-creation. Clean off your side of the street. Whether they reciprocate is up to them – just take care of your side of things. Breathe deeply and send love and *acceptance* towards the other party (rather than 'tolerance'). Remember that everyone is just looking for love and wants to be happy. Do what you can to help shift things back to a happy state. Be aware that the other person will ultimately either move into alignment with the space of love you are holding, or away. There are only two options if you really hold that space still, with sincerity.

Be Here Now

If you are going through a particularly rough patch emotionally and feeling surrounded by difficulties, try to gently bring yourself into the current moment and realise that right now, in this instant – which is really all you have – you are OK. Practice gratitude for *whatever* it is that you experience in each moment, the challenges as well as the joys. Yesterday your partner may have left you and tomorrow you may be facing eviction from your property, but right now, in this very moment, you can be at peace if you choose it. By dwelling on issues of the past or worrying about the future, you are simply giving away your power in the *present* moment. Breathe deeply, do not try to cope with more than one moment at a time, if necessary and reach out to others and Spirit for help (rather than food). You are not alone and you do not have to turn to food, to get through difficult times.

> ### Your Peace Candle Within
> One of my favourite tips for maintaining a peaceful state comes from motivational author Dr. Wayne Dyer. He recommends imagining a deep cavity within one's torso, in which is housed a brightly burning candle. This is our candle of peace. This candle represents the power within each of us to become present in every moment and feel serenity, regardless of what appears to be going on around us. Dyer recommends that in any time of stress, we turn our thoughts to this candle within and breathe deeply, keeping the flame burning steadily. Our aim at all times is for that light to stay burning strongly within, rather than getting 'snuffed out'. This can help us to feel relaxed, present, open and stable. I really love and appreciate this imagery and tune into it often.

Live Radiantly, Active Transformer *(Yes, that's YOU!)*

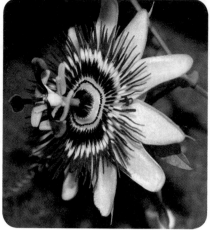

Whatever it is that you're doing, try to do it BIG. Give all your energy, focus and love into whatever it is you're engaged with in that moment. On an ultimate level, it really seems to make little difference *which* activities you're doing from one moment to the next – the *Universe* has no preference. However, doing whatever it is you're doing with a fullness of spirit, presence and love can make a huge difference in terms of positive impacts. So many people go through life with shoulders slumped, dragging their feet, mumbling or feeling like victims. Resist hiding your light and living small. So, for example, if you're rebounding on a mini–trampoline, make the jump bigger and more defined. If you're speaking to someone, be fully present with them, speaking clearly and audibly. There is truly an unending supply of energy in the Universe – tap into it, trust it and enjoy it for yourself. Make your impact in the world clear, passionate and strong and things will be reflected back clearly and with love to you too.

Rather than trying to do *everything* strategically in your life, be sure to explore your spontaneous and creative urges as well (perhaps even spend a day 'living by the dice' – throwing dice to determine your next moves). The Universe loves spontaneity and speed; it *literally* responds to your every thought and is ready in every moment to bring you exactly what your heart desires, if you trust, believe in it and allow it, rather than procrastinate. The Universe is always weaving **synchronicities** and clues into your path. Classic examples might be arriving at your destination in a car *just* as a parking space becomes clear for you to use. Or thinking of someone and he or she suddenly contacts you. There are no 'coincidences' in life– we are all connected and co-create synchronous events like this together. Try to be observant, watch for signs that the Universe is responding to your desires and flow with them, with faith. Many people find that the synchronicities in their life pick up pace as they go raw and get more in alignment with the natural rhythms of the Universe. You can choose to embrace the synchronicities and enjoy the unfolding ride, or you can block any offering as it arises. The Universe has no preference and will simply respond to *yours*. However, the more you DO flow with the synchronicities – and especially if you express enjoyment and gratitude for your experiences – the more will be at-

Paying Attention

I have intuitively sensed messages from 'Spirit' my whole life and the clarity of this communication seems to have increased in recent years as I journey through this healing raw transformation. The synchronicities and manifestations seem to become faster, clearer and more intriguing over time. Life feels like a more or less continuous flow of 'synchronicity' for me these days.

As a simple example, if I am trying to decide one morning what to do in terms of exercise and someone starts to talk 'randomly' about a wonderful hiking trail in the hills nearby, I take this as Spirit talking through that person and I listen and follow the prompt. Wonderful experiences tend to unfold.

A specific incident of communicating with Spirit that potentially saved my life occurred in Arizona. I had set up a little outside office space to work in, with cushions packed into a corner. One morning I came out to work and as I went to sit on the cushions, the small still voice inside me commented 'Maybe there's a scorpion under there...'. I was a bit sceptical but have learned to listen to that little voice, so I dutifully lifted the cushions to check for beasties. Sure enough, as I raised the pillow, I came eye to eye with the first scorpion I'd ever met. I smiled, breathed deeply and thanked Spirit for the guidance. It amuses me sometimes how 'indifferent' the resonance of that little voice can be; it certainly seems to watch out for my well-being, yet there is no drama attached to the outcome of any action I may choose. In this example, for instance, the little voice did not scream, 'OH MY GOD, watch out, don't sit there' – it just gently suggested that perhaps there was a scorpion under the cushions. The guidance can be very subtle and for this reason easy to ignore (especially for those in the hubbub of city life).

I do my best now to respond with speed, love and gratitude as things arise. However, sometimes I don't feel the courage to follow every prompt that is given and I may feel sad later if I sense that I've let something or someone 'slip through my fingers'. I know on an ultimate level, though, that it is all OK and this opportunity was just one in an endless field of opportunities. This 'blocking' is like procrastination on an energetic level - saying to the Universe, 'Hmmm...actually, I'm not quite sure I want to play out that experience right now' and side-stepping it for the meantime. I rarely behave in this way anymore: from experience, I've learned to flow with what arises, rather than resist and procrastinate. If I do push something away, though, I usually find that a very similar experience will present itself to me again on another occasion – a new opportunity to explore that particular energy pattern.

tracted your way. Life can become a **sensuous, flowing dance** of synchronous events.

New Frontiers

Transformation creates wonderful new vistas. Notice and enjoy the freedom you begin to experience through weight loss, such as any increased ability to participate in activities without fear and embarrassment. For example, you may suddenly feel motivated to attend a meeting in a local hall that you had always avoided because you know the chairs there are wobbly and likely to collapse under your weight. For those who have never lived with obesity, such considerations may seem bizarre, but for those living in obese bodies, the world can seem like a maze of potential embarrassments and difficulties through which to try to navigate. Freedom from such anxieties is therefore a real blessing.

Losing weight means adjusting to a new version of ourselves as part of our body disappears. This can be a strange and disorientating experience, as others may begin to react differently to us and we encounter new attitudes and expectations. We may find that having wished to

Coming Out of My 'Shell'

I remember how shocking I found the difference in peoples' reactions to me after losing weight. People everywhere seemed to treat me with so much more interest and respect. This actually raised up some bitterness in me, as I knew that I would have received very different responses just a few months prior; there was a lot for me to let go of, emotionally.

*I was shocked to find that men seemed to suddenly be looking at me on the street - I wasn't used to all this eye contact and felt embarrassed and vulnerable. Other women started to react differently to me too; I went from being the asexual, harmless fat friend to seemingly being viewed as 'competition'. My whole social world flipped inside-out and it felt very de-stabilising to me. Though in many ways it was exciting, I also felt quite lost and unprepared amidst these new social dynamics. I felt over-whelmed, for example, just **visiting** clothing shops: the petite shop assistants I'd always felt scared of were now being nice to me and I could suddenly fit into most of the clothes in the store. It felt like a different life...*

*I felt like I didn't know how to be the person that other people now seemed to think I was. I realised how much of a **protective cushion** my extra weight had been, in more ways than one. My fat role began to seem safe and cosy in comparison. Indeed, as a friend once pointed out to me, obese people rarely become presidents or leaders in our societies – it's simply not expected. Hence, staying heavy is one way to stay disengaged.*

*The **huge** social leaps that can follow weight loss are apparently one of the main reasons why many people who have released weight regain it again: consciously or unconsciously, the shifts seem too much to handle. However, I knew that I wanted to stay on the raw, healing path, so I breathed deeply and got on with it, using tips like those in this Guidance section to help me integrate all the new shifts and come up smiling.*

be thinner for years, when the change finally comes, we feel afraid. Food and fat may have been our escape route for so long that it feels uncomfortable to embrace the new and stop hiding our real selves away. Be gentle with yourself during your transformation and seek guidance from those who have had similar experiences.

The same can be true whether or not *weight* loss has been the main change for you. If your most significant transformation has been emotional, you may find that you now feel braver about going out in the world, yet also some-what apprehensive. Take this gently, expanding your 'safe' territory steadily.

Honesty

Say it how it is. Expressing your honest feelings to others with care, grace and integrity is a wonderful life skill to develop. As we've discussed, holding feelings inside where they can stagnate and fester does no-one any favours. Practice staying calm and centered in conversation, speaking from a place of truth within yourself. It definitely appears that the more genuinely honest we are in communication, the more our lives seem to effortlessly flow. This is not a suggestion to 'let rip' at others, however, with a barrage of opinions. Try to speak with compassion, love and acceptance when sharing your feelings. Say what you mean, without being mean. When you do have strong 'negative' emotions to release (such as anger) try your best to release that without directing it at other people. If you get the feeling that any attempt to speak your truth in a situation is going to result in a directed, angry explosion from your lips, you might try using one or more of the other tools here first (e.g. breathing deeply, pillow-punching) to diffuse the energy, before communicating your thoughts.

Do what you can to break down your barriers of secrecy and introversion. For addicts, there tends to be a direct link between secrecy and sickness. Make the effort now to reach out to others with your honesty and reveal who you truly are – the rewards will be manifold. Try to share **all** of yourself with people, not just what you consider to be the 'good'. Be honest about all that is going on for you. Vulnerability is our greatest defence. We are all human, fallible and in a constant process of change – there is nothing to be ashamed of or to hide from others. Simultaneously, as we share our truth, it encourages others to share theirs too.

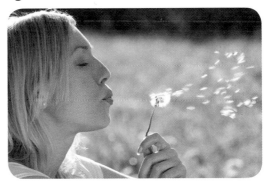

Detachment

A huge part of my own recovery was learning to *detach* from my co-dependent desire to do everything and be everything to everyone. What is 'detaching' and how can you do it? We can think about it as moving our focus and attention from an unhealthy emphasis on other people's activities, desires and wants, back towards focusing more on our own lives. Learning to detach *with love* was a big shift for me – i.e., not removing my love/attention from people altogether, yet respecting their freedom to make their own choices and do things for themselves. My co-dependent, learned patterns were wrapped up with control issues and fear – the (subconscious) desire to 'have control' over people and things in my environment. It felt like things were unmanageable if they didn't go the way I wanted. It took a lot of deep breathing and tears for me to let go. It feels wonderful now to be able to watch loved ones make their own choices from a distance, without trying to control any aspect of their experience. I can still be there to support and encourage them, I just don't try to do it all for them.

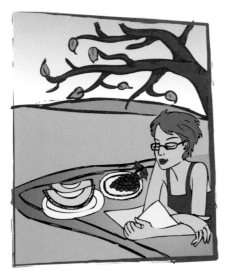

Values

A good way to establish real happiness and fulfilment is to examine your personal values. Make a list of what is really important to you. Then double-check if everything on this list is absolutely true for **you** or whether it is an idea you have 'bought in' from somewhere else.

What's on your list? Your health? Spending quality time with your family? Making time for yourself to do the things you enjoy? Next, take an honest look at the things in your life that you give most of your time and energy towards and see if these are the *same* things as you have written on your first list. This can be a really eye-opening exercise. We might well notice that the things which we claim to be of the highest value to us actually receive very little of our time or energy. Adjusting any imbalance between what matters to us and the attention we give it helps pave the path to a happier emotional life.

Moderation in All Things

We've heard it before, many times – but how well do we manage to sustain moderation in our lives? Many of us live with extreme internal landscapes. We're either fantastic or awful, gorgeous or pitifully ugly, 100% raw or bingeing on junk. Instead of this all-or-nothing, black-or-white thinking, we can balance ourselves out with some shades of grey (or better still, some rainbow colours!). 'I'm so much better/worse than you' can become 'I'm equal to you', 'I'm different to you', or even 'I feel no need to compare' – WOW!). It's all about finding the stable middle ground – a place of balance where we feel safe, happy and authentic. Life is not a competition. We can cooperate with others at all times if we choose to. There is really no need to compare ourselves to others – we are all on our own journey.

When we get into dichotomies in our head that we are 'completely' this or '100%' that, or when we make statements like we 'always' do this or we'd 'never' do that, we set ourselves up for potential stumbles. It seems like a far gentler approach to find and maintain a balanced place of open moderation, with leeway to flow in all directions, than to box ourselves mentally into a corner with no room for flexibility.

> *"Once the game is over, the king and the pawn*
> *go back into the same box."*
> *--Italian proverb*

Draw In Energy

Realise that you are a conduit for the Universal energy and that this energy is unlimited. Whenever you feel 'dragged down' and like you don't have any more energy to deal with something, breathe deeply and connect to that source of all energy flow, within you. I like to do this by actively engaging all my chakras, especially the heart and third eye. I call energy in, from my base chakra through to my crown, asking for my whole being to be filled with love, light and healing. I also use this technique while jogging or doing other exercises, when I start to feel tired – I call in extra energy, breathe deeply and press on.

Of course, you might not feel like pulling in more energy, for example, in the middle of a heated argument. It might be gentler to 'take time out', before privately calling in the energy to release and transform any toxic feelings you are holding. You can gather yourself back together and continue with whatever seems unresolved later, if desired.

Out of the Frying Pan...

As we come out of one addiction, we often start to slip into others, due to the compulsion to fill that gaping black hole within us. Therefore, be alert to any signs of developing other addictions in place of overeating/food addiction. Protect your emotional transformation. If you see other compulsive patterns developing in your life, examine the situation honestly and take action as necessary to strengthen your recovery. Keep in mind that all compulsive activity is indicative of a loss of connection to your true self.

Keep Filling Your Abundant Treasure Box:
A Bounty of Forty Healing + Tips

Congratulations! You've made it to the main Treasure Trove: forty tried and true, recommended activities to help support your transition into a life of joyful Maintenance and stability. All of these uplifting activities can be enjoyed instead of acting out your eating patterns. These tips help turn your attention away from eating, release the pressure and reinforce the realisation that eating is not the most important thing in the world. I recommend that you schedule some of these activities regularly, *as well* as spontaneously trying some out whenever you might be struggling emotionally or with cravings, or simply just feel like doing something new. You don't 'have' to do them all. No one thing is better than any other, so there is no order of importance in the listing. They are all gifts for your taking and you can pick and choose as you like, finding what works for you.

Just a reminder – give them a bit of a workout, to let the positive effects settle happily in, rather than rapidly dismissing anything.

Check Out and Review Your History...

Examining the patterns you grew up with in your family of origin can greatly help you understand more what shaped your development. For example, reflect on how feelings were handled in your family, or consider any addictions/patterns that others seemed to display. On reflection, does it seem as if you were spoken to honestly as you were growing up and really listened to? Was it 'OK' to talk about emotions? Is there a lingering sense that 'keeping up with the Joneses' and presenting a 'good' appearance was in some way more vital than honesty?

Were there any 'rules' you encountered about happiness in your family? Were you expected to appear happy all the time? Did you think that you couldn't be happy if others were sad? Were you scared of being happy? Write all these things down, even as brief notes, so you get a good overview and can refer back to it later.

Ask yourself in particular if you were 'allowed' to cry as a child. If upset, were you comforted, or instead ridiculed and shamed? Crying is an excellent way to release sadness – it is healing and healthy, whereas overeating is clearly not. If we let ourselves *feel* our sadness, it comes and goes quickly, whereas if we block it, then later wallow and cling to self-pity, the buried sadness can last a lifetime. Self-pity can be insidious: if we start feeling sorry for ourselves, our mind may jump at the opportunity to suggest that we 'deserve' something like chocolate or other 'Trigger' foods to help us feel better. Do

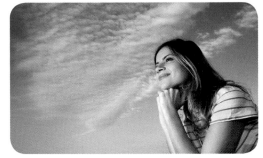

your best not to delve into pity parties, both when reviewing your history *and* in your day-to-day life.

We review our histories with the intent of releasing old feelings of guilt, shame and so on. We neither forget/deny the past, nor hold on to it with painful stories and feelings. We take an honest look at what happened, try to grieve any losses we feel, then put it all into perspective and move into enjoying the present. The past and future have no power over our enjoyment of the present moment, other than the power we give them by turning our attention and focus towards them. Do what you can to release your history with forgiveness and grace.

Many people also find it useful to enjoy a short, ongoing 'history review' daily as they go to bed. It can be very beneficial to think back through the day, giving gratitude for that which has passed and 'taking inventory' of anything that feels unresolved/uncomfortable for you. Perhaps you had an argument with someone, or felt very jealous towards a co-worker, or simply ate some things that you don't feel great about. Whatever it might be,

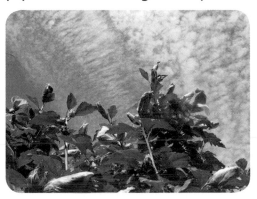

take an honest look at it, think about what might have been your motivation for behaving in that way and practice forgiveness, in whatever way seems appropriate. Over time, the more you focus on healing your patterns and shift into an increasingly loving space, you'll notice that these nightly reviews become less about resolving uncomfortable issues and more about feeling deliciously grateful.

Enjoying Time in Nature

I strongly believe that feeling disconnected from nature (whether consciously or not) is a major factor in
peoples' discomfort in our modern
societies. How many wild animals,
plants or trees do you have daily contact with? How many machines do you
have a daily relationship with? How
often in the space of an average day
do you actually touch the Earth with

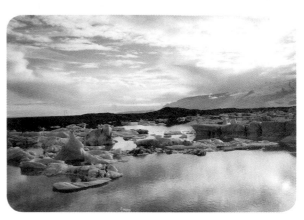

your skin? Our cities epitomise our disconnected cultures – people living
crammed in next to each other in air-conditioned, sky-high boxes filled with
manufactured material goods. We may 'pity' wild animals we see caged in
zoos, living their whole lives on concrete and yet many of us seem to *choose*
that way of life for ourselves. When you get to a new location, try to connect with it. Touch the Earth, say hello, eat something that grows there, if
you're able to identify edible foods.

If you are feeling troubled, try releasing your difficult emotions to nature
to absorb. Stand with your back against a mighty old tree and imagine your
issues being released into the well of wisdom, deep within that living structure. Walk with your bare feet on the Earth – a small patch of grass will do.
Or lie on the grass or a sandy beach and release your issues there. The power and strength of Mother Nature is infinite – she can help heal your pains.
Ask yourself this:

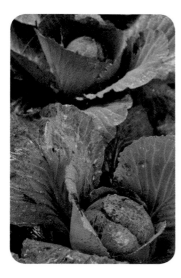

Which place on Earth do you find the most beautiful?

Chances are you almost definitely named a place out
in nature, right? A lake, a waterfall perhaps, your favourite beach, forest, mountaintop or field. Few people ever name buildings, highways, construction sites,
dams or railway bridges. (Incidentally, the place I find
most beautiful is featured in the picture above right
on this page – Jökulsárlón glacial lake, in Iceland.)
Enjoying time in nature is a fundamental way for us to
reconnect and feel at peace, away from the distractions of city hustle and bustle.

I fully encourage spending more time outside in natural settings, plus growing your own food. This is a wonderfully rewarding way to connect more to nature and also your own food source. There are few things in life so delightful as biting into produce you have raised yourself. Get your hands in the dirt and get connected.

(For books on growing your own organic sprouts and/or growing outside year-round, wherever you live, see the Resources section.)

"If you have a garden and a library,
you have everything you need."
--Cicero

Emotional Freedom Technique (EFT)

I was introduced to EFT by a dear friend, at a point when my life felt very much in 'crisis'. It is a superb tool and often felt like a lifesaver for me in order to get through that period. This simple and fast-acting technique is easy to learn. It involves tapping places on your body with your fingertips to release stagnant or uncomfortable energy and emotions in those circuits. EFT works with the subtle meridian lines of energy that run through the body, as used in acupuncture, although in EFT there is no use of needles - just your fingertips. EFT can provide relief for emotional discomfort of any kind - from handling food cravings, to road rage, to painful memories, to managing a broken limb.

EFT can be especially useful for those people who feel like they always have that 'last, stubborn ten pounds to lose'. Very often there are 'sticky' emotional reasons underlying this pattern, which go deeper than can be addressed simply through food intake and exercise. EFT can help us to address these emotional issues and finally release those last pounds. There are actually testimonies of people losing fifty pounds and more, *just* from starting to address the health of their *emotional* body in this way, without even making any changes to their food or activity levels.

One motto of EFT is 'try it on everything'. There is a basic tapping sequence to learn, along with a few accompanying things to say, to help focus your attention on the issue you're currently experiencing. All of this can be easily learned using the free manual that you can download at www.emofree.com. Another wonderful resource for EFT materials is www.TryItOnEverything.com.

Learning to Laugh Again

My transformation has helped me to 'lighten up' about life. After so many years of secretly feeling miserable, lonely and 'abandoned', I tended to take things rather seriously, as well as to isolate myself. A good friend said something to me one day that helped me shift my behaviour around this. He said that when he's around other people, he likes to have fun, because he can 'do the serious stuff' on his own. That really spoke to me. I'd been so serious for so long that it was like I'd forgotten to have fun with others socially. These days I prefer to reserve reflecting on and integrating the more challenging aspects of my life for my private, meditative times. This frees up my energy to enjoy being around others more and share fun in each moment.

Movement/Exercise

Being active is *the* way to get your endorphins flowing, release energy and feel great. Some of my favourite expressive ways of exercising are dancing ecstatically to music at home, 'Five Rhythms' dancing, rebounding, running and dancing with poi (spinning balls). Exercise can really help you to get out of your head and into your body, releasing pent-up emotions and feeling more grounded. The practice of yoga (which can be translated as 'union with the divine') is especially powerful for helping people to reconnect, relax and release. Yoga can be thought of as a dynamic form of exercise, meditation and prayer all rolled into one.

"What if the hokey-pokey is all it really is about...?"
--Jimmy Buffett

Eye-to-Eye Communication

'Real eye communication' is something I now love to share with others. This is the practice of keeping still and holding clear, constant, face-to-face eye contact with another being, allowing to unfold whatever unfolds. This for me feels incredibly healing, allowing each to bask in the pure meditative bliss of being truly seen and mirrored by another being, breathing deeply and connecting truly. No words, no pretences, just seeing another for the pure love they embody and allowing oneself to be truly seen at the same time. Bliss. (In some areas, you'll actually find 'eye-gazing parties' – definitely something to 'watch out' for...)

Sing It-Say It-Laugh It-Hum It

Our voices can be wonderful tools for self-expression. Laughter, humming, singing and even screaming are great ways to get energy flowing and to release emotions. Most people are aware of the value of laughter for healing and health. The average pre-schooler is said to laugh about four hundred times a day, whereas the average adult laughs about fifteen times daily. Enjoying more time around children might therefore be very healing for you – especially as we tend to laugh about thirty times more often when we're in company. Plus, if things are feeling a tad too serious, you could try transforming the energy by saying out loud how you feel in a 'Mickey Mouse' or falsetto voice. This is priceless for helping shift perspective and lighten the mood – so try it!

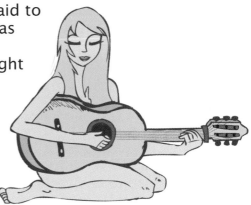

For me, singing is a great uplifter and form of expression too - I notice that when I'm truly feeling happy and relaxed somewhere, I start to sing. Some of the most serene and blissed-out moments of my life have occurred while participating in women's song circle groups, singing a cappella, or with hand drum/guitar accompaniment. Many of us regularly stifle and stuff our emotions and singing like this is an easy way to keep things moving freely.

Smiling and Having Fun

As the saying goes, 'smile and the whole world smiles with you'. It's not easy to feel negative when you have a genuine smile on your face. Simply put, smiling relieves stress. A smile shared with a stranger can have a positive impact beyond anything you may ever have imagined.

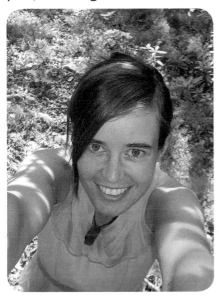

There's a tendency for people to get very serious while working through their emotional detox, especially at the beginning. Lighten up! Smile and remember that whatever *appears* to be happening on the outer is all ultimately a cosmic giggle and in truth, all is well. Choose not to take yourself or anyone else very seriously – a simple smile, shrug of the shoulders or laugh can be enough to disperse any collecting negative energy in a situation.

Do all that you can to nurture the beautiful, artistic, creative child within you who has been frozen for so long, as well as any zany, comical character you've been 'pretending not to be'. You wanna wear different coloured socks and angel wings today? Do it... You wanna go and play in a ball pit for two hours? Do it... We can learn to play again – to have fun simply for the sake of having fun - no justification, no competition, just plain creative fun. Participate in light-hearted activities that maybe you've denied yourself for years – laugh, enjoy and make time for leisure. An outstanding resource for learning to nurture the creative, spontaneous child within you is Julia Cameron's wonderful book *The Artist's Way* – see the 'Ten Books To Shape A Life' section below for details.

Gimme the Whole Works: Holistic Therapies

There are countless holistic therapies, courses and trainings that can help you get your body, mind and soul into better balance, such as Reflexology, Re-birthing, Polarity Therapy, Sound Therapy, Neuro Linguistic Programming (NLP), Acupressure, Reiki, Chakra Cleansing, Energetic Healing, Aromatherapy, Tantra classes, 'Journey' work, Colour Therapy, Theta Healing, Family Constellations, Vortex Healing, Flower Remedies, Psychotherapy, Gestalt, Float Tanks, Astrology Readings, Hypnotherapy and so on. Some are more body-based, some more 'head–focused'. Different therapies **resonate** for different people – you might want to test out a few at a holistic fair or wellness centre open day, for example, to see what feels good for you. Find a practitioner to work with whom you trust and feel comfortable around.

Retreats and Courses

Retreats and courses are a wonderful way to take time out from the pace and perceived problems of your everyday life. On retreat you can enjoy a relaxing, rejuvenating break somewhere with like-minded people. There are many different kinds of retreats available, from weekends to months, from silent meditative retreats to powerful inner-child workshops, couples healing, supervised fasts/cleanses, sweat lodge ceremonies and so on. Aim to go on retreat yearly for at least a week. Or you might choose to do an invigorating weekend course on something like Non-Violent Communication, foraging, storytelling or windsurfing. Whatever you choose, these times are optimal opportunities for breaking up and releasing old patterns (especially food-related), as you're away from your familiar structures and routines. Many people who struggle with going or staying 100% raw by themselves find it useful to go on a fully raw retreat somewhere, so that they are immersed in that lifestyle for at least a few days. This can make all the difference in terms of shifting patterns. Enjoy!

Get Creative

If you're feeling an emotional block, try releasing it through a creative – rather than destructive – medium. It's time to get solutions-orientated and focus your energy on *projects,* rather than '*problems*'. You might paint a canvas, write some poetry or pen a letter (maybe you never send it – just getting the stuff out of your head is beneficial). It can feel very cathartic to channel

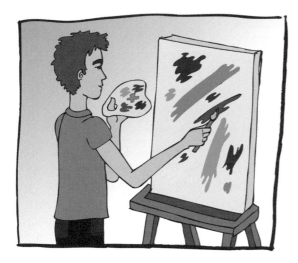

your energy in such a positive, constructive way. Afterwards, you might feel relaxed, relieved and have a piece of art to share as a result, rather than a fiery shouting-match of emotions followed by silence and pain! When engaging in such an activity, try not to use it as avoidance, however – consciously focus on releasing your angst as you create. In this way you will free yourself rather than simply suppress the emotions for a while, which may then re-emerge at another time. Of course, you can always paint a joyful painting too, if that's what comes...

Counselling

When we go into active transformation work, it might feel very dramatic in the first few months, when lots of raw emotions are coming up. There may be masses you want to express. You may feel that, even if you have explored many of the avenues described here for releasing your emotions, there is still more that you want to say that you don't feel comfortable sharing with those in your life. It can be a great relief for all involved if you seek out a counsellor of some kind to speak with regularly. The tidal waves of emotions we experience as we shift can put a great deal of strain on relationships, especially if you are bubbling up with lots of resentment, bitterness and tears. Rather than perhaps relying on the same people to fill all roles in your life, finding a counsellor to express yourself to can provide an amazing, impartial outlet for your releases. You may feel more able, especially in the beginning, to share some of the more painful things being released for you with a 'stranger' like this than with those to whom you are more intimately connected. This person's *job* is to listen to you, after all, so you know you definitely have their attention, plus they likely have a great deal of experience to draw upon, to give you guidance and perspective.

Resting and Relaxation

Many of us lead very fast-paced, hectic lifestyles with myriad commitments that keep us in an almost constant state of tension. We may feel like we're strung out, always tired and 'never get time for ourselves'. If you're literally finding yourself falling asleep while doing tasks, it's time to re-evaluate. Relax. Slow down. Recognise that how you use your time is *always* a choice. Take an honest look at the activities you take part in: do you really feel it serves you to be involved in them all? Are there things you could lay aside and instead catch up on some much-needed rest? Remember that the resting is as important as the doing.

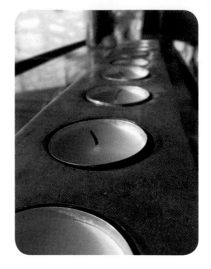

When we feel great *ourselves*, then we are in an optimal position to serve others. It is most beneficial for everyone concerned if we take care of *ourselves* first. Again, many *women* especially give their power away in relationships, over-extending and putting other people before themselves moment after moment after moment. Soon enough they're feeling strung-out, filled with resentments, tired and miserable.

Try to simplify your life so that your **commitments** are fewer and instead create new, nourishing, relaxing rituals for yourself, like a weekly deep soak in a bubble bath, for example. It also helps to ensure that your house is uncluttered, peaceful and feels like a sacred space in which you can relax. When we are deeply relaxed, our brain waves slow down into the alpha or even theta states (rather than the usual day-to-day beta state). The alpha and theta states involve slower brain wave frequencies and seem much more effective for creating positive, healing shifts in our lives. (For more info on brain wave states, see the Resources section.)

'What Happened?'

If you find yourself in a situation where you feel upset, angry or uncomfortable and you can't seem to shift that feeling, try to get very quiet within and ask yourself 'what happened?' What series of events or actions resulted in you feeling unhappy? Treat yourself as you might a young child you come across who is crying or frustrated. Become the observer, extending compassion, comfort and understanding to yourself. By gently asking 'what happened?', we can begin to contemplate the events leading up to our current situation with more objectivity. This is like taking a step back from the situation and simply recounting what unfolded, impartially, without exaggeration, blaming or drama. This is usually a *great* help for seeing a situation more clearly or opening up a different perspective. It helps us get out of a stuck head-rut in our current moment and start realising solutions instead. The chances are high that, as a child growing up in our modern Western cultures, whenever you were feeling unhappy, the expression of your feelings was not strongly supported or mirrored. You now have the opportunity as an adult to support *yourself* in taking an honest, clear look at what is happening for you emotionally.

Acts of Service

A fantastic way to get out of your own 'story' is to reach out and support someone else.

When we are isolated in our own thoughts, patterns and perspective, it's easy to go in negative circles in our heads focusing on 'problems'. Get out of your head and into your heart, with thoughts, words and deeds centered in love. Become solutions-orientated and focused on what is beneficial for all – for the community. If even one person in that community is hurting, it affects the whole – you can reach out and offer support, no matter how beset with issues you may feel yourself. Don't wait until you feel 'well enough' or 'good enough' to give. Help others and contribute to your own healing by reaching out and giving. Even if 'all' you offer is a smile, a shoulder to cry on or a genuinely listening ear, these are all potentially enormous gifts from the heart and can help you to put your own 'issues' into perspective.

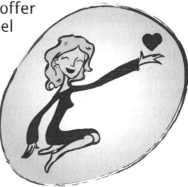

It is especially effective to include in your prayers those whom you sense are currently ill or weak in their energy. Picture them as being well and happy – send light, love and healing energy towards them. All that we give out to others with love is returned to us manifold – so step past any thoughts of 'lack' and share your best today with someone whom it seems would appreciate some support.

Thank You, I Love You, Please Forgive Me, I Am Sorry

One of my favourite ways to dissipate awkward energies and painful emotions is to share these four blessings: thank you, I love you, please forgive me, I am sorry. You may recognise this as the Hawaiian healing process of 'Ho'oponopono', which is based on loving yourself and accepting responsibility for all that is within your reality. There is a wonderful story that accompanies this prayer. One ward for the 'criminally insane' in the State Hospital in Hawaii was home to those patients who had been declared more or less 'untreatable'. A healer went to work there. He never met with any of the patients. He simply went and sat in an office and read over their medical files. As he read, he felt loving compassion and blessed each of them repeatedly with the healing prayer: 'thank you, I love you, please forgive me, I am sorry.' The transformation in the patients was remarkable. Their conditions shifted to such a degree that in the end, the hospital ward actually closed, as there was no longer any need for it...WOW! I love that story – for me it totally conveys the message of the power of our thoughts. So, next time you feel anger, disappointment, jealousy or resentment towards others, perhaps try saying this prayer – either out loud or internally - and watch the energy transform... You can find out more about this simple healing technique in the Resources section.

Sound It Out – The Healing Power of Sound

Ever wonder why we talk of people being in *sound* health? Never underestimate the power of music to help people shift things and heal. Whether you put on some Mozart, R&B or drum 'n' bass to soothe your soul, the results can be tremendous. Music touches parts of us that may not otherwise seem accessible and can help us release things that may otherwise stagnate. Perhaps in a dark moment you pick up a crystal bowl and its gentle tone soothes you, or you pump out an Alanis Morrisette CD in your car's music player and sing along at the top of your voice while driving. Whatever it is, notice afterwards how your mood has transformed merely by connecting to the energy of the music. One of the pieces of music I find the most calming is the 'Tat Tvam Asi' devotional singing CD from India that we have for sale in the RawReform store. This was recorded by friends in the eco-city of Auroville in India and there is something very peaceful and inspiring about this piece for me – it especially helps me to concentrate. Tat Tvam Asi was in fact the 'soundtrack' for me almost exclusively as I wrote this book; I had it on loop in the background, helping me to stay focused.

Positive Thoughts and Words

This could be considered **the** key for transforming your life. Thoughts

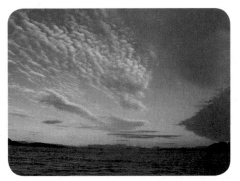

are things: so choose them with care! Your thoughts and words are extremely powerful. In fact *all* that you create or manifest here begins with thought. What you **think** about, you **bring** about. If we really appreciated the power of belief and positive thinking, it seems unlikely we'd ever choose negative thoughts. Yet so many of us go around in circles of negative thinking in our head. We judge things as 'bad' or 'wrong', talk about how we 'hate' people/things, discuss what we see as 'problems' and so on. If you understand that you are **creating your own reality**, moment by moment, ask yourself this: 'What do I want to create now?' Do you want to perpetuate misery, disappointment and fear, or would you like to live in the light of love, joy and gratitude? Choose your thoughts and words with care. I strongly discourage using words such as 'bad', 'wrong', 'evil' and so on, as these all tend to carry a heavy 'negative' energy. What one person considers wonderful, another might think outright awful. It is all a matter of perspective. Where do you want your energy to be directed?

Try this exercise: for the first hour of the day, try to only speak if you have something positive, generous or

What Do I Love?
The following is a list of things I enjoy in life - you could write one of your own...

I love to sing, dance, bike, jog and rebound. I am a poi/fire dancer. I have been in many musicals and other stage shows. I love interacting with animals, sharing photos with people and reading. I find it very rewarding to build a strong network with other women, wherever I go. I love challenging myself. I adore both giving and receiving massage – it feels very sacred to me. I like gazing deep into another person's eyes and asking them what they're most afraid to tell me. I thrive on the truth.

I look forward to skydiving one day, as well as travelling in a hot air balloon. I enjoy learning more about foraging and anticipate attending a raw permaculture course, to prepare for starting my own gardens somewhere. I love the sun and warmth.

I tend to collect small things everywhere I go - especially stones, feathers and shells. I collect songs in my head - I think the biggest part of my memory banks are composed of song lyrics...

I am a money magnet - I have always found money and other dropped items, since I was a child. I take every single penny as a sweet gift from the Universe. I collect together too the magical stories of people whose lives are transforming as they embrace more vibrancy through raw foods. As I live on the road, my physical possessions are not so numerous or large – that keeps life simpler and lighter for me.

uplifting to say. Notice how this affects your outlook and experiences.

"If you are irritated by every rub,
how will you be polished?"
--Rumi

If you notice that your thoughts and words seem to be 'negative', you can breathe deeply, express that you are sorry, forgive yourself and then shift your focus to something positive. Worrying about things also does not serve anyone positively. Choose not to think and speak like a 'victim'. Replace limiting thoughts of failure and lack with visions of success and prosperity. Write out a gratitude list for everything that you have already experienced for which you feel grateful and revisit/add to it whenever you feel a tad less than grateful. Practice living with an 'attitude of gratitude'. More will be attracted to you as you focus your attention on that which you love. Whatever we put our focus on expands. What would you like to have more of in your life?

Post Up Your Joys! Another simple way to keep your thoughts, words and deeds positive is to surround yourself with uplifting messages throughout your home. In your bathroom, for example, hang an inspirational note near the toilet, or use post-it notes to stick up messages, or an eyeliner to write love notes to yourself on your mirror. Help yourself to stay motivated and positive.

Engaging in transformation work is surely one of the most positive things you've ever done for yourself, so enjoy it. Notice all the changes that you're experiencing with your feelings and your interaction with others and recognise the gifts of health you're giving yourself and also others around you. Weed out any ongoing 'stickiness' in your thought patterns; consider for example how much time you may actually spend focusing on what you feel you've done 'wrong' with food, rather than celebrating all the steps forward you've taken. If you find that you seldom focus your energy towards your highest vision of yourself, ask yourself how could this be redressed. Help maintain your positivity by staying away from 'negative' people and worrisome situations, especially until your own emotional boundaries are strong and well-developed.

(One tip that helps *some* people to maintain a positive focus is to imagine that you are pregnant – yes, women often resonate more with this suggestion than guys. Wouldn't you prefer that baby to develop inside you surrounded by loving, positive, supportive

Is it 'You', 'I' or 'Them'...?

I recommend taking 'ownership' for your own feelings and experiences, particularly as you speak. When many people speak, they generalise the topic away from themselves by saying something like 'You feel rejected when someone doesn't like your ideas', when the real meaning is 'I feel rejected when someone doesn't like *my* ideas'. If we regularly use this kind of 'distancing' with language, it is less easy for us to be aware and present with our emotions and experiences, because we're always 'projecting' them away from ourselves. Create clarity in your expression and 'own' your feelings as you speak. If you mean 'I feel/I want/I am', then say 'I' rather than 'you'.

A similar pattern occurs when people speak vaguely about 'they/them', referring to some undefined group of people, often inferred to be opposed to 'us'. Examples might be 'They keep raising the cost of living', 'How can they let someone get away with that?' or even 'They say Italy is beautiful in spring'. This lack of clarity leaves questions hanging in curious minds: who are '*they*'? How did 'they' become something different from 'us'? Where do the opinions and actions of this invisible 'they' come from? This kind of expression reinforces an outdated, separatist model of 'them vs. us', often with some sense of victimisation and oppression, rather than an understanding that we are all connected. I usually sense these speech patterns as disempowering and unclear. Speaking with integrity and clarity of expression, rather than in vague, generalised terms, will assist your alignment with truth; it can help you feel more secure in your self and more aware of what you perceive. Be clear about what *you* think and feel and who 'they' really are.

thoughts? Wouldn't it feel rather toxic and unpleasant to be having negative, judging, miserable thoughts streaming into that being, as it grows in you? Now consider that your *own* body and tissues are affected just as powerfully by your thought patterns. Do you really want to keep 'poisoning' yourself from within like that?)

Pilgrimage

If you are seeking to really disconnect from your current patterns, you might find it beneficial to go on a pilgrimage somewhere. This might be on a path commonly known for pilgrimages, like the Santiago de Compostela in northern Spain, or it might be any trail that feels sacred to you. You might go alone or with others; you might even choose to walk in silence. Pilgrimages are a time to disconnect from any apparent external issues we have been experiencing in life and turn our reflection inwards, healing ourselves and the whole as we journey. It can be a miraculous time of transformation and feeling connected to source. (I recommend the books *No Destination* by Satish Kumar and *Peace Pilgrim* by Peace Pilgrim for inspiration on pilgrimages.)

Your Dream Map

A fantastic creative way to brighten up your thoughts, outlook and imagination is to make collages of the life you would LOVE to be living. Gather together a pile of old magazines and newspapers, scissors, paper and glue (or a pin-board and pins). Simply flick through the publications, looking for pictures that appeal to you as part of the life you'd love to be living. Maybe it's an image of a house you find beautiful, or a wonderful beach, trees, a happy family, a calm lake – whatever appeals to you. Arrange the pictures on either a sheet of paper or the pin-board and fasten them. Keep this posted somewhere visible in your home so that you can frequently see it and draw inspiration. You might want to do various collages for different aspects of your life – your health, your body image, your finances, your primary relationship and so on.

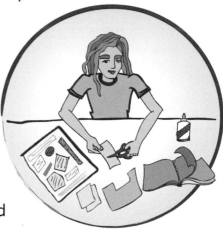

Innertalk CDs

Innertalk CDs use subliminal messages to impact the subconscious mind of listeners and help re-form their perspective. When played, the CDs sound like either nature sounds or classical music, yet beneath the 'surface' flows a constant stream of human voices sharing positive, uplifting messages. These messages are absorbed by the subconscious and can then start to positively impact your life. They are reported to be especially effective when played as you sleep. This is a very simple, cheap and effective way to see results. There are many different titles in their range, from 'Joyous Day' to 'Freedom From Junk Food' to 'Ending Procrastination' and so on. See the Resources section for more info.

Watching Films

If I am feeling very emotionally wrung out, 'lost' in my head or really need a

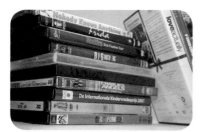

break from my own thought processes and perspective, I watch a film. Films are a kind of therapy for me in this way, as I lose myself in *someone else's story*. I get out of my own apparent drama. I also love films because in the space of ninety minutes or so, I get a whole story. That doesn't seem to come so easily in any other form and it gives me 'closure'.

I don't own or watch a TV, so watching films these days feels quite bedazzling to me. I allow myself to get completely drawn into the images and story. By the end of the film, my mood and perspective have almost inevitably shifted. Of course, I choose films that help shift me into feeling good.

It almost goes without saying – yet I'll say it anyway, just in case - that it's wise to be vigilant about what you feed your consciousness. Watching violent dramas, sarcastic, caustic comedies or news programmes full of fear are unlikely to serve your optimal well-being. Choose light, uplifting or educational films. Some of the films that have most inspired me are: *Raw For Life/Simply Raw*, *Birth As We Know It*, *The Secret*, *Conversations with God*, *What the Bleep Do We Know?*, *SuperSize Me*, *Amelie*, *Life of Brian*, *Rabbit-Proof Fence*, *Try it On Everything* and *Whale Rider*. (The Spiritual Cinema Circle provides a wonderful selection of entertaining and inspiring films. The site TED.com also hosts a free, fabulous selection of short, inspiring talks from some of the 'greatest thinkers' of our times. See the Resources section for more info on these.)

Your Divine Diary

Keeping track of your experiences by writing them down is a fabulous way to get an overview of what is really happening for you. It gives you something to refer back to later on, to track your process and see how far you've come. Also, if it appeals to you, this can be something to share with other people who are transforming *their* lives. You might want to keep a hand-written journal, or you might prefer to write on a typewriter or computer. Blogging is a popular modern form of online journalling. Anyone can create his or her own blog (derived from the words 'web log') online for free and start recording their experiences. Popular sites to use are www.blogger.com and www.wordpress.org. The RawReform E-Journal can be seen at http://rawreform.blogspot.com. I write there usually every other day or so, recording my Food Plans along with all kinds of musings on raw food and life in general. I love blogging, as to me it feels like 'writing an email to the world' and I also love to look back at old posts and see how things have shifted in my life. There are many raw food blogs out there now. It can feel very exciting to start sharing your thoughts with the world and getting comments and feedback. You can even make your blog private if you prefer, so that only registered users can see it. I encourage blogging for both creative outlet and feeling account-able – living your life out in the open and with integrity. The more people who are out there in the world sharing their truth about raw food and transformation, the easier it is for us to spread this healing message faster.

Sharing Circles

I highly recommend seeking out others who resonate with the experiences you're having, to share together in a group circle setting. An issue pondered in isolation can seem immense, whereas sharing that same issue with others who understand, may help make it seem not only manageable, but also easier to transform. Ideally in such groups each person gets the chance to speak their truth as they desire, without interruption, feedback or judgement. It is a safe environment in which to share openly. Many such groups already exist, such as Overeaters Anonymous, Co-dependents Anonymous, Al-Anon and so on. (These are all '12 Step' groups, in the tradition of Alcoholics Anonymous, as previously mentioned.) Find other **Active Transformers** who 'have what you want' in terms of emotional health and find out what they are doing to build and protect their boundaries.

There are also many independent healing circle groups you can find. One

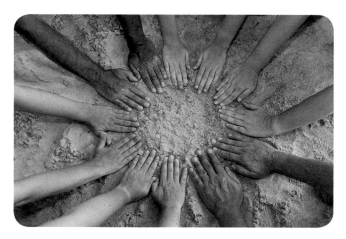

group that I thoroughly enjoyed in Connecticut, for example, is called The Passion Project. It is a women's meeting group with roughly thirty attendees and every week, one woman shares about *her* passion in life, for approximately forty-five minutes, with time for others to share afterwards. I love the positive focus of that group.

Look for something that offers *ongoing* support, to keep your connection and motivation going. You may also consider setting up a group yourself if there are none in your area. Even initiating an 'inspiring reading circle' with a couple of friends can be the start of your own supportive community. There are also *online* and telephone meetings, which are great if you live in an isolated place or want to be part of a meeting at a time when you know there is nothing happening near you. Groups such as Overeaters Anonymous for example have regular phone meetings and online meetings conducted in 'chat rooms' – see the Resources section for more information. Often, as our lives begin to transform, we sense that things are different and yet do not find it easy to articulate with confidence these changes, or how we feel about them. Attending meetings where others on a similar path are talking about their experiences can be a great benefit in this regard. You can pick up new ways to relate to yourself and others, plus 'get out of your own head' as you listen to others' stories.

If you're thinking to yourself 'I don't have *time* for meetings', consider the following tip from self-development writer Melody Beattie: There are 168 hours in each week and taking just one or two of those hours for sharing your feelings in group gatherings can help you maximise the potential of your remaining 166 hours. Meetings can act as release valves, helping to bring your life into a space of **greater serenity** and joy, rather than passing time worrying, complaining, obsessing and so on.

Another easy way to connect to other people who share your interests, at any time of day, is to join online community websites. We are so blessed to have the internet to help us connect now; in the twentieth century, most raw foodies felt a lot more isolated. Now we can reach out easily to connect with others all over the world.

There are a few popular sites for raw foodists, where you can 'meet' new people and share ideas in a more informal way than at meetings. Examples at the time of writing are www.TheRawFoodWorld.com/ic and www.GiveItToMeRaw.com. Other great places to look for online raw friends are the community on RawReform.com, MySpace. com and Tribe.net. The site rawfood.meetup.com is also wonderful for finding info on raw potluck gatherings and meeting others in your area. (You can start a new group if there are no meetings yet in your location.)

Meditation
There are many different types of meditation techniques that all assist in helping us return to our natural state of being. Meditation is nothing more or less than focusing your attention on a single point – perhaps your breath, a part of your body, a mantra or something similar.
You might associate meditation with monks in caves or monasteries, yet people all over the world, in every walk of life, use meditation as a valuable relaxation tool.

Meditation is easy to learn. In fact, many people frequently experience meditative states of some sort in the course of simple activities like walking in nature, or performing tasks such as raking up leaves. It is about being in a state where the normal internal chatter of our minds is quietened and we find ourselves instead in a more contemplative place.
In truth, there is nothing extraordinary about meditation – it is our most

natural state. It is the calm, blissful condition of a baby, for example, or any animal at rest in the wild. In our societies, we seem to have become so 'disconnected', piling so many complexities into our lives, that we frequently find ourselves in a befuddled maze in our heads, anxious, stressed and far from serenity. Engaging daily in meditation is a way to heal that rift.

One of the most important things to be aware of when starting to practice meditation is releasing any perfectionistic expectations of how it 'should' be. Don't try to force any outcome or over-analyse your 'success' – just enter the process and observe what happens.

Mellowing into Meditation

For a long time, I had big mental blocks about meditation. I told myself it was something for other people, that I 'just couldn't do it', that I didn't have the time/patience/money to learn it and so on. These days such thoughts are long gone for me and meditation has become a central part of my morning ritual. The change for me came very simply – not by attending any expensive course, finding a 'guru' or spending hours learning to meditate 'properly' – I just decided to give it a real chance. One day I simply began to sit in a quiet place, legs crossed, back straight for ten minutes, attempting to connect in my own way to the still small place inside me, which blends with Great Spirit. It worked – afterwards I found I felt calmer, more connected and at peace, so I continued with this practice, day by day. Gradually over time I discovered that the moments when my mind was quietened and I was focused simply on 'being' started to outnumber the moments of mind–chatter. This was very gratifying.

I feel large energy surges as I meditate and a great deal of love. I see this part of my daily practice as the part where I am 'listening' to the Universe and Spirit, rather than talking and asking (prayer). I offer myself as a conduit for the energy of the Universe to flow through me and show me its will. Sometimes I am given key insights for the unfolding of the day or future ventures in those moments. Sometimes it is more like a clean flow of loving energy, filling my being with healing. I try to be still and present, listening to any promptings of the Universe as I would listen to the talking of any friend – with an open perspective. Aside from a focused meditation session like that each morning, I also re-focus into meditative states throughout each day, especially whenever I feel uncomfortable, anxious or fearful. Meditative states come naturally to me now, while walking, playing, communicating and so on - without any focused action of sitting and going into that space. By putting aside my hang-ups about meditation and just giving it a try, I opened up for myself a whole new world of peace, calm and serenity.

(If you want to learn more about meditation, you might like to read some of Osho's books, such as *The Book of Secrets*.)

Find a quiet, comfortable place to meditate and ideally position yourself with your back straight, either sitting or lying down on your back. You do not have to be cross-legged. Begin with meditating for a short time, perhaps ten minutes. Focus your attention on something, be it a colour, an object in front of you, a mantra or your breathing and try not to harass yourself with expectations of how long you must stay focused – staying focused for longer periods of time becomes natural with practice. It is not about concentration, effort or endurance; it is rather something effortless and truly refreshing. If you find your attention has drifted to other thoughts, simply observe this and move your attention gently back to quietness – think of these 'interruptions' like passing clouds. Daily practice of meditation techniques is very beneficial for relaxation and reconnection to your inner voice.

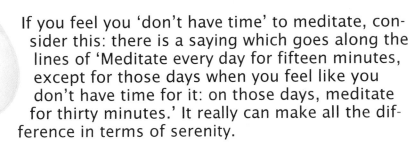

If you feel you 'don't have time' to meditate, consider this: there is a saying which goes along the lines of 'Meditate every day for fifteen minutes, except for those days when you feel like you don't have time for it: on those days, meditate for thirty minutes.' It really can make all the difference in terms of serenity.

Affirmations/Inspirational Cards

I like to draw a card from an inspiring deck every morning. The cards have beautiful affirmations on them like 'I am willing to forgive', 'It is only a thought and a thought can be changed' and 'I say YES to life'. Affirmations are statements that can help us increase the power of positivity in our lives and raise our self-worth. They help set an uplifting tone for my day. I leave the card I've picked for the day on display, so that I see it and am reminded regularly of its message. I encourage using these little 'touchstone' packs to help brighten your day or share with others– they make wonderful gifts. We sell packs of inspirational cards in the RawReform Store.

Aside from such cards, people often write out affirmations, or repeat them – either in their head or out loud – perhaps while looking in a mirror. There are many different approaches like this for helping to shift our thinking into a more positive space. You might like to consider affirmations such as:

I eat only nourishing raw foods.
I love every part of my body.
My detox is gentle and steady.
I love my food choices.
My healing is unfolding at exactly the right pace for me.
I am worthy of love and recovery.

My feelings and needs are important.
I feel healthy, vibrant and enthusiastic.
I am loveable, loving and loved.
I have the right to be myself.

For best results, keep the words and focus of your affirmations positive (i.e., avoid phrases like 'I mustn't, I can't, I don't' and words like 'bad, unfair, painful' and so on). Also ensure that your affirmations are something you can really believe and feel good about – e.g. if you are currently three hundred pounds, choosing the affirmation 'I am one hundred and twenty-five pounds, slim and agile' may seem totally distant and unreal to you, whereas 'My body is at a healthy weight and I feel active and energetic' might work. Everybody is different and affirmations that work for you may hold little appeal to someone else.

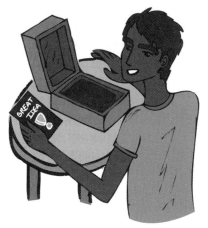

Slogans
There are many supportive slogans we can use as gentle daily reminders for our path. Here are some commonly used in 12 Step Programmes:
· Progress, not Perfection
· Easy Does It
· An Attitude of Gratitude
· Misery is a Choice
· One Day at a Time
· Just for Today
· First Things First
· Fake It Until You Make It (to positively condition yourself into any behaviour you find hard to adopt initially, such as really accepting and loving your body.)

Writing these slogans out and carrying them with you, or putting them up on post-it notes in prominent places are effective, simple ways of actively transforming your everyday life. (Pssst, if you sneak a peek at the end of this book, you just might find a special free gift along these lines, waiting there for you to enjoy...)

Deeeeeeeeeep Breathing

Deep breathing is of the utmost value for your health, happiness and emotional stability. It is often the quickest route to serenity in any situation, plus it's easy and it's free. Many people's breathing is shallow, only filling the upper third of the lungs. When we breathe deep down into the diaphragm/abdomen, it helps to relieve stress and also supports the lymph system. Check in with yourself during the day and see how your breathing is going. Try to consistently breathe more deeply and slowly.

To me, deep breathing feels like calling in extra support from the Universe. I visualise the breath flowing into me with white light and radiance, helping me relax and filling every cell and part of my being with light, love and healing energy. There are many breathing techniques you can learn: a well-known therapeutic practice is Qi Gong, which incorporates different breathing patterns with physical postures. One of the greatest methods for deep breathing that I have learnt in recent years is Holographic Breathing, taught by Buddhen in England – for more info, see the Resources section.

Open to Serenity

A simple prayer that is commonly used in both 'recovery' circles and by many individuals throughout the world is known as 'The Serenity Prayer' and goes like this:

'Grant me the serenity,
To accept the things I cannot change,
Courage to change the things I can
And the wisdom to know the difference.'

Saying this prayer can provide great **relief** in times of discomfort or conflict. It helps us to release our will to control *everything* – such as other peoples' behaviour and choices.

Prayer

Whereas I see meditation as a form of 'listening' to the Universe, I view prayer more like 'speaking'. I connect to Spirit and express my intentions and desires. I affirm that I am a conduit for the Universal energy today and want to act from a space of love, for the good of *all* oneness, everywhere. I want to step away from actions that are chosen primarily to serve my ego. (In meditation I may then receive some feedback in the form of images and so on.)

I would love to share here my own prayer, which developed in me over time in the mornings as I awoke (I no longer use this prayer personally, yet it was a great touchstone for me during the period in my life when I engaged with it daily.)

Hi God, Hi Spirit...
I hand my will and my life over to you today,
For your care and keeping.
Make your will mine, I choose your will as mine.
Please make me want to do what you want me to do,
I choose to want to do what you want me to do.
Please guide me through the day, showing me each step along the way.
Guide me away from:
Fear, animosity, self-hatred, judging, blaming, expectations, self-pity, self-ishness, lack of connection, criticism, anxiety, resentment.
Guide me towards:
Love, honesty, connectedness, truth, serenity, peace, joy, sharing, expression, creativity, wonder, spontaneity.
Make your will mine. I choose your will as mine.
On the basis of my recovery, may others realise the benefits of being close to you.
May thy will, not mine, be done,
On Earth as it is in Heaven.
If it is for the good of all oneness, everywhere.
Amen.

The parts where I asked to be guided away from certain things and towards others changed each time. I used whatever came to mind in that moment on that day. I feel that 'God'/Spirit's will for me (as for everyone) is simply to enjoy my experiences and act with love towards all. That is what I ask to be guided towards with this prayer, rather than anything self-serving/strongly ego-based. I feel that praying in this way first thing in the morning helps establish a solid connection with Spirit from the offset and declares the will to surrender ego that day.

In prayer, I feel that it's a great idea to preview our plans for the day, ask for inspiration, intuition and the power to act in a way that is for the good of all oneness everywhere. Then we can let go and get on with our day – we've said where we'd like to go today, now get in the passenger seat and let the story unfold by itself, rather than trying to control the details. (Personally, I use a much simpler version of the above prayer these days. I basically express my intention to act as a free-flowing conduit for the Universal ener-

204

gy, ask for support with that, give thanks and think about how I'd love to see the day unfold. Then I let go.)

Visualisation and Goal-Setting

Take the time every morning to visualise your day. I do this each morning during prayer. This helps focus my attention on the things I love and enjoy and gives a direct message to the Universe of those things I would like to experience. I take a few minutes to overview the structure of the day – the things I would love to experience – along with a general 'slideshow' in my mind of what I find uplifting. This 'slideshow' might include things like laughing with friends, receiving wonderful news, cuddling, rolling down grassy hills, jumping on a trampoline or whatever comes to mind. This doesn't necessarily mean that I want to experience all of those things *today* – it just helps me to be in a positive space and attract more enjoyable experiences. I find visualisation like this a wonderful practice, to help me stay focused on what feels good to me and I enthusiastically recommend it to *you!*

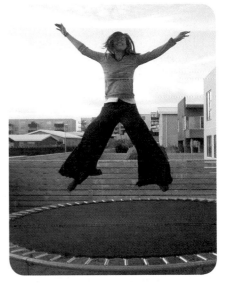

On the bigger scale, making a list of your goals - things you want to experience in life – is another great exercise. Your list might include anything from 'move into a brighter home' to 'get a massage once a week' to 'visit Japan'.

Personally, I write out a list of things I intend to experience as life unfolds and then keep the list safe. I see it as my 'order' from the menu of life, which, of course, carries every 'dish' available. I make my list, then let go of it and take my attention back to the present moment. Our thoughts are **extremely powerful** and I know that once I've made my 'order', it's more beneficial to let the Universe do the unfolding in its own particular way, rather than 'chasing after the waiter' and checking up constantly to see if he's fixing my order exactly the way I'd choose...

Some people refer to this as 'letting go of the HOW'. Just be clear about what you'd love to experience, then let go of HOW that is going to manifest in your life – let the Universe work its magic. This does not mean being idle, however, sitting back and expecting everything to fall into your lap. You can still take *action* towards the goal, just let go of *fretting* about how this goal will be realised. Keep your faith in the bigger picture while taking steps forward daily, following the path as it unfolds.

It feels best to me to state my *preferences* in life, but not to try to control the outcome. I sometimes visualise whatever I have 'requested' as a beautiful, blossoming flower, starting to unfurl. If I then become over-eager to see the end result and try to peel open layers of the leaves and petals before the flower is ready to reveal itself, I may ultimately sabotage its development or perhaps even destroy it. My sense is that the best I can do for anything I 'put out there' is just to nourish it with the vibration of pure, unconditional love – no strings attached, no conditions, no expectations, just love and gratitude – and trust what blooms…

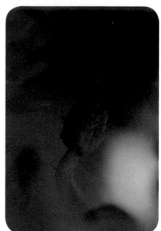

Goal-setting on the grander scale and visualising on a day-to-day basis are like getting your road map/directions for where you want to go. Of course, you *can* do things and get places without a clear plan, yet why would you want to, when you could take a few moments to get things clear and shape your own delicious journey? Where do you want to go? What do you want to do? *Write it down*. It can be considered 'just a dream' until you write it down, then it becomes a *goal*, a mission statement for your highest vision of yourself. As the writer Anaïs Nin put it: 'If it's not written down, it doesn't exist'.

Then to reach that goal, let go and retain an unswerving belief that it is all coming to you, just as you outlined. By committing to a series of action steps, you will see your goals realised. Ask yourself: what is the *very next action step* I can take to realise this goal? Is there a certain person to call? An email to write? A drawer to open to find a certain document? Whatever 'comes' to you as the next necessary step, **do** it.

Releasing
A fantastic way to dissipate and release pent-up frustrations is with some pillow-punching. If strong, heavy-feeling emotions are with you – anger,

resentment, bitterness, rage – you can stack up a pile of cushions, pillows and blankets, focus on whatever issue or emotion is concerning you and then release your feelings straight into the pillow pile. Simultaneous screaming, shouting, crying and vocal expression while punching can really help move the energy. You may want to warn others in the vicinity before you start releasing. I'd recommend that you keep up the releasing until it feels like the energy has gone out of the situation for you, or you've tired yourself out. It's also great to meditate afterwards, to settle back into a more serene space and really feel the difference in your energy body after the release.

Juice Feasting

I encourage Juice Feasting as a way to disconnect for a while from your emotional ties with solid food and get perspective. Your relationship with food might be seen like any 'sticky' relationship – when you're tangled up in it, it is not easy to see clearly what is happening. Juice Feasting brings the time and space to take a **healthy break** from those endless emotional eating circles and form a new approach for your relationship with food, post-Feasting. It's not necessary to Juice Feast for 92 days (like I did) to feel this kind of shift – even *one* to three days of straight juicing can be time enough to get a good break from compulsive habits. Or perhaps you might enjoy making one day every week your 'juicy day' and drinking only fresh raw juice on those days? This is a great way to give your digestive system a weekly rest. If you want to know more about Juice Feasting, please see my book *A Juice Feaster's Handbook*, which is available from the RawReform site, or visit JuiceFeasting.com.

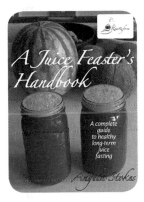

Crystals

In recent years, I have come to appreciate more and more the healing power that certain stones and crystals seem to bring into my life. I like to visit crystal shops and find stones that really resonate for me when I look at or touch them. I have a slowly growing collection of stones that I really love. I carry them with me everywhere I go, in a small pouch, along with other little 'treasures' that hold positive energy for me – like pieces of jewellery, feathers, sticks and so on. I connect in with these objects at times when I feel discomfort and it soothes me. I also very much appreciate the presence of healing crystal salt lamps in homes and the beautiful tones of crystal singing bowls.

You might find it very beneficial to create a little 'altar' in your home or work space, where you can gather together any crystals, pictures or other objects that hold value for you. Connecting to this space can help you to 'recharge your batteries', relax and feel more connected to Spirit.

Next time you are near a crystal shop, you might like to pop in and simply pick up and hold any stones that appeal to you. Some stones are considered to have a specific healing quality, but a great way of finding ones that work for you is just by holding them and seeing how *you* feel.

Touch/Massage

Loving touch heals. Sharing physical touch with others has been an important part of my healing process. As an obese person I felt 'untouchable' and was physically isolated for many years, starving myself of contact. Although I was actually desperate for contact and intimacy, I was so disgusted at my own body that I wouldn't accept contact with others, even if it was offered.

In my healing, massage and bodywork have been vital tools for helping to reconnect to both others and myself. As it turns out, people say I'm a 'natural' at giving massage – I really enjoy it, as a kind of meditative practice, connecting with the essence of another and helping to relieve their blocks. I also love to receive massage – it helps me to let go of things. When I first

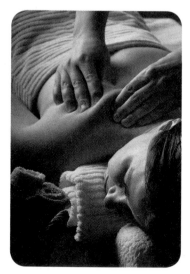

released all that extra weight, I was very 'jumpy' if people touched me – I just wasn't used to it. I had to let go of old ideas that it was unpleasant for others to have contact with me. Sometimes these days I'll still shudder or recoil a little if touched, yet overall I've moved happily into feeling comfortable with touch. There are MANY different kinds of massage – I would recommend choosing one of the more 'healing' varieties, such as Shiatsu, Hawaiian Lomi-Lomi or Deep Tissue.

I feel that *many* people in our societies are touch-deprived (especially those who are obese) and that this can have a big impact on health and happiness. Most people know that babies deprived of human touch and contact often die very young (e.g. in mass orphanages). Imagine that same impact on adult humans, on a widespread scale. We are all looking for love. Try reaching out to someone today who you think would appreciate a hug or gentle arm squeeze. It's amazing the difference that touch can make for healing pain and bringing people together.

If you feel very uncomfortable about the idea of physical contact with others, it's a helpful practice initially to place your *own* palm on, for example, your leg and simply experience the feeling of the palm of your hand on your own skin for a few moments. Or try stroking your own cheek or forearm, or even as a preliminary practice to resolve traumas around touch, begin to gently use a dry skin brush. These exercises can help establish the feeling that physical touch can be pleasant and nourishing. Gradually, we may start to feel more relaxed about having physical contact with others.

(There are actually now 'Cuddle Parties' regularly organised in many big cities. These are sex-free, safe environments for people to lie down and cuddle together, enjoying human contact. See the Resources section for more details.)

'I Love You's

Whether thought, written or spoken, every word affects the whole in some way. The vibrational power of words cannot be underestimated. You might, for example, be familiar with the *Hidden Messages in Water* work by Masuro Emoto, which shows us how the physical structure of water can change according to the **vibration** of different messages sent to it. I believe the same goes for everything (yes, even apparently 'inert' objects such as computers, washing machines and cars, to a different degree). One exceptionally simple approach for positively impacting those around you is to practice saying 'I love you' (internally or out loud) to everyone and everything you interact with throughout your day. This can feel an especially powerful thing to do, for example, as a form of walking meditation while strolling down a street. Practice sending a message of 'I love you' from your heart chakra out to each person or group of people you pass. You may choose to focus extra love and blessings towards people who appear to be in distress: a crying child, an angry teen, a weary mother. We are *all* connected; all love that you give out comes back to you manifold and your loving messages to the world help brighten all experience. Share some of the good juju today!

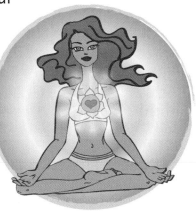

Non-Dominant Handwriting
This is a very simple technique to deal with any deep

blocks you may have, especially with your beliefs. It helps us to tap into different neural pathways and step outside the usual framework from which we see the world – our 'dominant' **perception**. We do this simply by writing, using our non-dominant hand. For right-handed people, use your left hand for this exercise; and left-handed people use the right hand. If you are ambidextrous, use whichever hand you tend to favour less. This is ideally a two-stage process: first writing about how you *currently* feel towards something, then writing about how you would LOVE things to be.

Let's say (for example) that you feel uncomfortable about your relationship with and understanding of 'God'/Spirit. Spend a few moments getting focused on that issue. Then, taking a pen, pencil or crayon in your non-dominant hand, write out how you feel about this relationship. Try to keep your language simple and your thoughts clear - let your feelings flow. You might like to draw a picture too, to illustrate your thoughts. Then on another piece of paper, write about the kind of relationship you'd LOVE to have with a Greater Power – feel free to draw pictures here too if you like. If it feels good to you, you can then scribble out the writing on the first page – be sure to do the scribbling with your non-dominant hand too. This helps to release that old energy. Some people also like to tear up or burn papers like this, in ceremonial fires, as a way of releasing.

What Would LOVE Do Now?

This is a pertinent question to ask yourself, especially in any situation that feels uncomfortable, to help shift the energy. Stop, breathe deeply and ask yourself, 'What would LOVE do now?' Right now, what is the most loving, generous and open-hearted action you could take? What would be your highest vision for the outcome of this situation? By focusing your energy towards these positive thoughts and solutions, rather than staying stuck in whatever feels unpleasant, you can help turn a situation around. Rather than sitting in a victim role, blaming someone else or circling in resentments, we can release that energy, with love. There are few things as beautiful as witnessing the feeling of love in the space where once there was pain. Of course, use of this technique doesn't need to be restricted only to times when you sense tension – you are free to spread love in *all* moments!

These days, if I find myself with some spare 'down time', I use it to concentrate positive, loving energy and thoughts towards others. I also visualise the things I love and enjoy in life. This seems to me like the most beneficial use of my energy in any given moment.

Treats

As you 'transform', treat yourself to a lot of love and attention, with *non*-food items. You'll most likely have more money to be able to do such things now that you are not buying junk foods. Perhaps you'll buy that necklace you've been admiring in the shop window for weeks, treat yourself to a day at a spa or send yourself a letter in the post with congratulations on your ongoing transformation. Work out what feels nourishing for *your* emotions and helps you build your recovery, rather than eating. Your inner child **loves** this kind of fun, by the way, so tune into what feels like it would be exciting and nourishing for you to enjoy and *do* it, preferably at least once a week.

Check in with yourself too about your concept of food 'treats'; is it possible that you're still thinking of cooked cakes, fried prawns or buttered toast as a treat? Is there a lingering notion of 'on a special occasion, I'll 'treat' myself to a cream cake' or something similar? If so, ask yourself if you really want to be living with that kind of world view, or if perhaps the idea that refined sugars and other processed foods are a gift to the body might be a little out-dated and could be released...

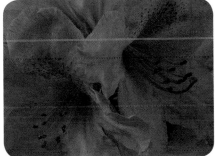

You might like also to consider the words of Jeanne Calment from France, the longest-lived human on record. Jeanne died in August 1997, aged 122. In her later years, she commented: "I took *pleasure* when I could. I acted clearly and morally and without regret. I'm very lucky." There's a saying that 'success leaves clues' and I think this is great guidance from Jeanne: go for the pleasure, treat yourself (and others) well and enjoy the ride. Incidentally, Jeanne also apparently attributed her longevity and relatively youthful appearance (for her age) to olive oil, which she reported using on all her food and rubbing into her skin.

Automatic Writing

This is a very simple way to connect to the messages from your deeper self. Find somewhere quiet, take a pen and paper and sit calmly, breathing deeply, getting centred. Focus on any issue you would like more insight into and then, as you feel inspired, start writing down on the paper the messages that flow from within you. Some people find it challenging to do this exercise, as it involves 'switching off' the analytical part of us and letting answers flow from within. Your writing ought to flow freely and effortlessly – this is not something you *think* about. You are not rationally answering any question, correcting grammar or anything of the sort. Your writing is free-flow and 'automatic' – you may not even understand what you're writing as you write 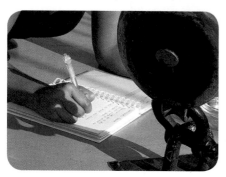 it – that's OK. You may like to write using your non-dominant hand for this exercise too, to further access 'hidden' parts of yourself.

When the energy to write has dissipated, you might like to then take a breather before reading over what you wrote. Some fascinating insights can be discovered this way. You may be completely amazed at what is written before you and wonder 'where' it came from. It is simply the Universal flow of energy, working through you. Some people also get sceptical and confused, concerned about whether they're 'just making it up themselves'. The way I see things, we are all connected, so whether something can be said to come from 'just you' or 'just' anybody else seems like a redundant concern. If it is something *useful* to you, then surely that's all that really matters? Try to drop the head-space and just enjoy the experience, with gratitude for what has been shared.

Inspirational Audio

There is an absolute wealth of information available in audio formats these days. Listening to educational CDs/MP3s while driving, exercising or doing housework can open up many new doorways for you and is usually a much quicker way to access info than reading books. One audio set I love is from **David Deida**, who speaks about relationships and communication. I have listened to many of his CDs. Listening to his work on masculine and feminine energies helped me to get more clarity about the dynamics in my own relationships. I also really appreciate the work of Caroline Myss, who speaks about archetypes – e.g. the child, the victim, the saboteur parts of us – and the effects of these archetypes on our choices in life.

I highly recommend subscribing to PhilosophersNotes.com, which hosts a fabulous collection of 'mini-Cliffs Notes for self-development books'. The notes are accessible in both PDF and MP3 formats and offer wonderful condensed insights into some of the most inspiring books available. See the Resources section for more information.

Ten Books to Shape a Life

There have been many books in the last few years that have helped guide me on my path. Here I'm going to share a little about ten of the books that have had significant impacts on my emotional and spiritual path. I recommend having inspiring books like these easily to hand, so that whenever you feel a little down, you can open a book at a random page and read something uplifting.

Non-Violent Communication (NVC) by Marshall Rosenburg

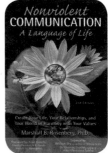

This outstanding book opened huge doorways into my heart. Rosenburg outlines a simply wonderful technique for communicating with others from a place of honesty, integrity, responsibility and compassion. Training in NVC can be accessed worldwide.

Homecoming by John Bradshaw

Healing and supporting my 'inner child' is an ongoing process for me. Like so many people, as I began to examine my patterns in life, I discovered a very hurt, frustrated and sad 'child' inside me. Nurturing that child aspect of my being is vital for my happiness now. One of the books that most helped me to examine and integrate this part of my life was *Homecoming* by John Bradshaw. This has a workbook format, with many wonderful exercises to help guide you back to a more loving and integrated relationship with yourself. His book *Healing the Shame that Binds You* also helped me a great deal.

Daily Readers

These little books contain insightful, motivating, uplifting texts and thoughts for every day of the year. I recommend keeping them by your bedside or in the bathroom for a daily dose of inspiration. The benefits of reading one short page can stay with us throughout the day. I bought mine from recovery specialists Hazelden, who have many different titles – from *The Language of Letting Go* to *Food for Thought* to *Easy Does It*. Hazelden also send out free daily inspirational emails delivered straight to your inbox, called 'Gift for Today', which is a nice way to start your mornings – see the Resources section for more information.

The Artist's Way by Julia Cameron

This is another book that had a profound impact on my life. In fact, you would very likely not be reading *this* book if I had never read *that* book! *The Artist's Way* inspired me to quit working in a job I really didn't enjoy and to start writing my first raw food book. I felt encouraged to take the creative leap. I came to realise that my misery in the job I was doing served no-one. I trusted that I would be carried in this venture, if it was truly for the good of all oneness everywhere. Well, it certainly feels like I received that support!

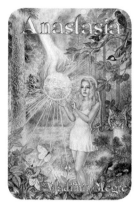

Anastasia by Vladimir Megré

The 'Ringing Cedars of Russia' series of books have affected me more than any others in recent years. Megré's real-life accounts of his meetings with Siberian forest-dweller Anastasia are simply spellbinding for me. I find the richness of Anastasia's connection with the whole web of life incredibly inspiring. To me, she represents a modern-day powerhouse of truth, light, integrity and beauty.

Conversations With God by Neale Donald Walsch

This series of books had a profound influence on my life during a period of much torment. Reading these books helped me to release a great deal of anxiety, blame, fear and resentment and to move onwards in life. The simple, accessible truth shared in the conversations between the writer and 'God' touched me deeply. During some of my darkest moments, reading these books felt like my lifeline.

Mutant Message Down Under by Marlo Morgan

This is the anecdotal account of one modern American businesswoman's encounter with an Aboriginal tribe in Australia. She thought she was setting out with them for an afternoon 'walkabout'...many months later she emerged from the bush, with extraordinary tales to tell of all they had shown her about reality from their perspective. Fascinating stories of connection, nature and perception shifts.

The Law of Attraction by Esther and Jerry Hicks

In recent years, the Law of Attraction concept has become quite widespread, especially due to the popular film *The Secret*, which shares similar information to this book. This is a channelled piece of work and I found that it imparts some very useful life tools, especially concerning visualisation. This

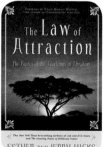

book helped me a lot with releasing negative thought patterns and instead creating solid, positive intentions for my reality.

The Power of Now by Eckhart Tolle
This classic of our time is another book filled with such profound simplicity that virtually every sentence strikes a chord of truth somewhere in my being. I feel like just opening this book relaxes me – I know that no matter which page I open it to, there is going to be something there to enlighten, uplift and help centre me into the present moment.

Raw Family by The Boutenkos
This is the simple little book I read in May 2002 that kick-started *my* raw journey. It's a very inspirational, quick read that offers the Boutenko family's testimony of how their lives completely shifted after going raw. As their illnesses receded, they set off walking the Pacific Coast Trail, from Mexico to Canada, with many adventures along the way. They've since inspired countless thousands into improved health. A wonderfully uplifting book.

Stack Your Shelves

There are many other books that have also helped me on my path, in some way or another. These include (in no particular order):

Bliss Conscious Communication by Happy Oasis (Fabulous guidance for free-flowing, fun conversations.)
Peace Pilgrim compiled by Friends of Peace Pilgrim (Available for free as an e-book or hard copy, in many different languages from http://www.peacepilgrim.com.)
A Course in Miracles scribed by Helen Schucman (Find *your* path to inner peace.)
Gaviotas by Alan Weisman (The story of an inspirational intentional community in Colombia.)
Love Without End by Glenda Greene (A beautiful, deep-reaching, channelled interaction with Jesus.)
Alcoholics Anonymous - The 'Big Book' by AA Services (The original recovery handbook.)

*__The Road Less Travelled__ by M. Scott Peck (Another detailed self-help classic.)

*__The Five Love Languages__ by Gary Chapman (Excellent book for learning to relate with your loved ones in meaningful ways.)

*__Learned Optimism__ by Martin Seligman (Fascinating insights from a world-renowned psychologist on how we can *choose* to be optimistic.)

*__Chicken Soup for the Soul__ by Jack Canfield and Mark Victor Hansen (Wonderful collection of short, inspiring, heart-warming stories.)

*__No Destination__ by Satish Kumar (The magnificent autobiography of the wandering ecological pioneer.)

*__Co-dependent No More__ by Melody Beattie (Good for addressing co-dependent dynamics.)

*__Healing the Child Within__ by Charles L. Whitfield (Great overview of inner-child work and addiction from a leading self-help author.)

*__The 12 Steps To Happiness__ by Joe Klass (Small, very insightful guide to the 12 Steps.)

*__Theta Healing__ by Vianna Stibal (Learn more about how the frequency of your brain waves can assist your healing.)

*__Personal Development for Smart People__ by Steve Pavlina (A unique book that gives a structured, practical overview of effective 'self-development' for all areas of life.)

*__Shelter__ by Lloyd Kahn & Bob Easton (Beautiful, enormous volume from the '70s, with more than a thousand pictures of handmade, eco-friendly homes worldwide.)

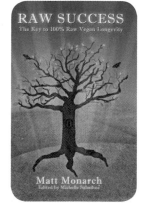

*__Become Younger__ by Dr. Norman Walker (The detailed insights of a remarkable raw food pioneer, reported to have lived to at least ninety-nine years old.)

*__Raw Success__ by Matthew Monarch (For in-depth info on staying healthy at the physical level over the long term, as a raw vegan.)

*__The Secret Life of Plants__ by Peter Tompkins and Christopher Bird (Phenomenal insights into how plants sense and interact with their environment, including human thoughts.)

Maintaining Maintenance

So, you've made it through the ups and downs of the Transitional stage - finding out what works for you in terms of healing, taking positive action, working through the major emotional bumps and, who knows, maybe even eating more raw food...? ...and now you find yourself gently living in a balanced daily rhythm of Maintenance; your emotional connections with food feel joyful again, you are genuinely happy with your life and most of the time you feel content, serene and loving. You are an exemplary Active Transformer... What now?

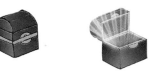

To continue enjoying a happy Maintenance, here are ten key tips, to use as you choose:

1. Continue to use a daily **Food Plan**, if this serves you. This usually helps hugely in staying on track. If you hit a sticky patch with your Maintenance and feel tempted to drop everything and reach out for your old Trigger foods again, consider that it is much more complex to *regain* your position 'on the wagon' than to simply maintain your stance there. If you come from a background of food addiction, you'll know that overeating is not actually an easier way of living (though your *mind* may try to suggest that). Overeating may give a superficial feeling of joy for a few moments; however, ultimately, it is destructive, multiplying issues for us rather than helping us move into more serenity. Lovingly preparing and following a daily Food Plan that you feel good about is a very simple way to stay on your healing path.

2. Practice a sense of calm and balance about *tiny* details. If, for example, you eat one more slice of cucumber than you'd intended to, there is no need for that to equal a 'relapse' in your recovery. However, *obsessing* about that extra slice *may* end up destroying your serenity, should you choose to believe that it *does* constitute a relapse and that therefore everything is ruined and you may as well just give up and eat anything. Try to keep things in perspective, be gentle with yourself and choose not to create drama around your food choices.

3. Keep your focus away from taking that **first bite** of a Trigger food, which seems to invariably lead to another and another, sometime soon after. As Overeaters Anonymous texts share, there's no need to worry about all those other 'bites' of food if the *first* one doesn't happen.

4. Keep dipping into your alternative menu of diversions – the 'Treasure Box' you now have holds many different ideas and activities that you might focus your attention towards instead of food. Keep this book somewhere handy (not tucked away in a drawer) and revisit the Guidance section often, for fresh inspiration.

You have a choice in every moment. This new path may not always feel easy, yet it's certainly healthier than the manic world of compulsive overeating or patterns of eating to suppress emotions.

5. Keep hold of some 'before' pictures of yourself, to take a look at now and then for inspiration. You might also want to read back through old notes/journals, or watch old videos of yourself, as a reminder of where you came here from. You are doing **great**.

6. Keep your 'Optimal Vision' handy. Whenever you feel inspired, check your current lifestyle against the one you outlined at the beginning of this book as your Optimal Vision for yourself. Make any manageable adjustments necessary for a closer or exact match. Also take a look at the 'Emotional/Spiritual Checklist' at the end of this section for extra reflection. Use this to validate and celebrate your successes so far in leaving aside foods and patterns that no longer serve you.

7. One practical point to consider in terms of maintenance is to keep checking and re-checking food labels for 'Trigger' ingredients. Listed contents can change and many products that may claim on the front to be 'sugar-free' or 'lite', for example, actually contain common Triggers, so stay vigilant. Remember that MSG (for example) is frequently passed off with terms like 'natural flavourings', 'spices' and so on. If you notice that your moods or health are strongly shifting and you can't pinpoint why, check the ingredients on any pre-packed things you've been eating recently – you may find some clues.

8. If you don't already have one, get yourself a companion 'Raw Emotions' fridge magnet from the RawReform store and stick it up on your fridge as a daily reminder that 'The answer is not in the fridge...' You could even use

it to post up your Trigger/Vigour Lists, Plan of Eating or Treasure Box list - oooo la la! Remember also to check out the last few pages of this book to locate your special, inspirational surprise treat...

The **ANSWER**
is *not* in the fridge... ;)

...try reading
'**Raw Emotions**'
instead...

www.RawReform.com

9. 'Holidays' and social events can feel demanding in terms of staying on track, even for those in Maintenance mode. Indeed, many people find it much easier to feel good about what they eat when they're preparing and eating food just for themselves. As soon as other people come into the picture, it can seem as if the *boundaries* slip around more easily and it's possible to lose track of what it is that **you** really want to eat. This is another example of how having a daily Food Plan can be a tremendous help. If you've chosen a plan for that day of what you're going to eat and you follow it, you can easily feel good, even if you are around others who may be eating differently. It can be useful, especially near the start of a raw transition, to be sure that you prepare foods on holidays that feel special to you, as these occasions are frequently based around food. If you sense that you will feel 'left out' in some way, you can create culinary wonders of your own instead, so that you *all* feel great.

10. One unusual tip to stay on track with moderate eating is to use cars less often... This might sound odd at first, yet if you try it out, I think you'll agree that if you transport your groceries by bike or by hand as you walk, there is less tendency to buy and use excessive quantities. If you're accustomed to filling your car up with groceries, I suggest that you try biking or walking your produce home for a week; see how it affects your outlook on what you use and consume. I find that this tends to make a significant difference in peoples' consumption rates, as well as (of course) helping reduce pollution, increasing the exercise you are getting and many other benefits.

Similarly, growing your OWN produce can encourage moderation too, as it helps you feel much more connected to your food source. For example, the first strawberry of the season from your *own* berry bushes seems so much more precious somehow than a box of shop-bought fruits. Foods we grow ourselves, with love, tend to inspire more respect and moderation in us – we usually want to savour and enjoy them, rather than wolf them down.

What To Do If You 'Slip' and Eat Things You Didn't Intend To?

Whatever the reason for the break, there is no reason to *panic*. Breathe deeply. You can get back on track at any moment. What happened has happened and there's no changing that, but you can affect what happens next by getting back to your Food Plan for the day, as soon as possible. One slip does not have to equal a slide into toxicity. Don't *give* up because you had a *slip*-up. You have a choice in every moment.

Try not to blame, shame or judge yourself for the break and avoid thinking in terms of having 'cheated'. If you make a 'mistake' and go off your plan, it doesn't mean that you *are* a mistake. Often, we find that we learn more about ourselves from our 'slip-ups', so choose to look on the positive side. See results instead of failures; you did what you did and it produced results. Considering that you are free to choose how you perceive that result, why not pick a description that helps you feel good?

Practice forgiveness with yourself, talk to others about what has happened (if you find it beneficial), reflect on whatever it shows you, then try to let it pass and get back on track. Holding onto the event with fear and shame serves no-one positively. Remember that transformation is about progress, not perfectionism.

Since we have clearly learned that uneasy feelings are almost as toxic as the processed foods themselves, if you *are* going to eat that croissant, at least LOVE and appreciate the experience. You can get back to a more optimal nutritional intake later. Fretting about your food choices does you no favours.

If you've eaten something that's particularly toxic for your body, such as a fatty hamburger or sugary cake, make sure that the next meal or two that you eat are as **high raw** as you find comfortable. Drinking a green vegetable juice is also great at this time for helping to re-balance your body. All this will give your body extra help in sweeping out the toxins from the junk foods and you'll ideally get back on track faster. Apparently apes do exactly this. If they've eaten something dense, which causes fermentation, they follow it with very fibrous foods to sweep out any mucous build-up.

If you're feeling *especially* jaded after eating other-than-optimal foods, a round of colon cleansing can also thoroughly help relieve the stress on your body, along with a generous helping of digestive enzymes. (Please take careful note: these are suggestions for 'emergency' handling of any rare occasions when your body has become uncomfortably unbalanced, rather than recommendations for *regular* practice.)

Remember that recovery is always there, always available to you - you just have to reach out for it and take action. If you are in contact with a sup-portive group, you will find no judgemental voices condemning you if you 'slip'. You will find love, acceptance, understanding and hope. You don't have to live in regret or fear about going off track. Try to live simply and peacefully in the *current* moment and enjoy your incredible transformation.

You can be confident that it also gets progressively easier to not pick up toxic foods or overeat, the longer we're off the highly processed stuff and following a regular, balanced plan. The processed stuff just doesn't look like food anymore and loses its appeal. Many people actually report that if they've been eating raw for a while, then try one of their old 'favourites', expecting it to taste just like it used to, they discover that it now seems like cardboard in comparison to fresh raw flavours. So, sometimes apparent 'back-step' experiences like this can actually *help* people to move away from cravings, as they realise they simply aren't interested in those old favourites anymore.

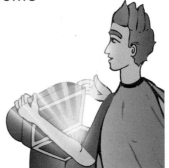

Remember too that you now have your personal Treasure Trove of supportive transformation tools and tips to dip into, to help get yourself back on track. Use it!

Enjoy Moderation

I want to highlight the simple and important overall message of seeking moderation, balance and consistency in our lives. We're looking for long-term health, rather than instant gratification. We're tuning into and supporting the part of us that wants the best for ourselves in the long run. This isn't to suggest that we neglect our happiness and enjoyment in the *present* moment – we just aim for supportive, consistent choices that over time add up to a balanced life. Rather than following knee-jerk responses to every 'demand' of the addict in us for distraction – 'I want this hamburger', 'gimme another double gin' and so on – we can slow down, stay centred and calm and make gentle choices.

It seems to me that consistency is one of the main things people struggle with in life, in all areas. It seems like a huge challenge for us to choose something outside our comfort zone, then steadfastly and *consistently* include new and positive behaviours. (Incidentally, have you ever considered the irony of the term 'comfort zone'? We tend to use this phrase to describe territory that we feel is 'safe' or even 'sensible'. Yet often this 'safe haven' of habits does little to genuinely serve our well-being. Could the term 'comfort zone' in fact be a common paradox...?)

Balance and consistency are major keys to feeling happy, solid and serene in the long run. There may be days where we suddenly enjoy a piece of apple pie that we would no longer regularly choose to eat. That's OK; from the bigger picture, it's what you do MOST of the time that counts, not the little 'blips' here and there. However, if your 'blips' seem to be getting so frequent that they could almost be mistaken for Morse code, it might be time to re-evaluate your situation! Aspire to experiencing genuine consistency most of the time – rather than repeated cycles of random compulsion and regret – and you will be on track to live a long, happy and healthy life. Many people find it easier to be consistent by making *small* adjustments, little by little, rather than trying to flip their whole lives inside-out overnight...

"What wound did ever heal but by degrees?"
--Iago, Othello

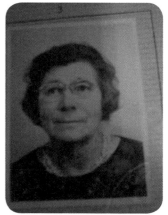

My grandmother Lily lived to be almost ninety-six years old (here she is, pictured to the right, aged sixty-four in 1970). She was not a raw foodist, although she did grow her own produce, like many women of her era. Lily ate what could be considered a 'standard' British diet of the twentieth century. She could also often be heard to say 'A little of what you fancy does you good'. I believe this simple outlook on life and nutrition to be one of the main reasons she lived so long. This was no complex philosophy based on scientific research. Lily just lived a life of simple, happy moderation. She seemed to understand intuitively that eating *anything* to excess was harmful to the body, yet *denying* oneself something that the heart desires is detrimental too. She took **the middle path**. She consistently ate small amounts of whatever she felt good about and thrived. I have a great deal of respect for the path she walked and her simple message.

Now imagine the impact that simplicity could have on one's life *while* eating mainly or exclusively raw food! Wouldn't *that* feel like a blessed, vibrant, healthful way to live? That's what excites me. It is not something beyond anyone's capabilities. Once we get the most toxic foods out of our systems and are 'in the zone' with a raw food life-style, *any* of the food choices we make are likely to be more healthful and supportive. With a raw food lifestyle of small, regular meals, we can create ongoing resonant health. Indeed, perhaps if my grandmother had been a raw foodist, she would have lived even longer and almost certainly she wouldn't have lived with the degenerative diseases such as Alzheimer's that she experienced in her final years.

It's important to remember that overeating *anything* is detrimental to health, regardless of whether it's raw or not. A raw binge can certainly have less of a dramatic impact on the body, compared to a toxic processed food binge, yet the strain on the body from dealing with a large load of food is never pleasant. Overeating also affects lifespan. Any animal that consistently eats small amounts will experience more longevity than those who overeat on large meals.

Eat less, live more.

Beyond just what you eat, try to integrate balance and moderation into all areas of your life. As previously noted, my life used to be full of extremes. With reflection, life, as a result, felt very dramatic and imbalanced for me. It was draining to live in a landscape where everything was a self-created drama and obstacle. It seemed like if I did anything, it was to excess. I exhausted myself with my 'perfectionism', rushing from one task to another – studying, volunteering, working, socialising – while constantly feeling stressed that I wasn't doing things 'well enough'. I am very happy to have slowed down since then and moved over to creating balanced days for myself now. My life as an Active Transformer is composed of a bit of meditation, a bit of yoga, a bit of communicating with people, a bit of quiet time, a bit of reading and so on: little bits of lots of things go to create an enjoyable, balanced day for me. This feels like a much easier, effective and calmer way to realise and live a productive and balanced life.

Here's a word of warning... When you do get to a point where you're in a happy state of Maintenance, feeling balanced and consistent, you might just find that suddenly...it all begins to feel a bit boring... Where is the drama now? What is there to fret about or distract yourself with? Where is the entertainment? An irony of the healing process is that often, when we actually reach that steady place we so longed for, it seems dull. We might find ourselves reaching out towards other things/activities/compulsions for 'entertainment' instead, consciously or otherwise. The human mind is almost always looking for distraction; it loves it. Just be aware of *what* you're reaching for...try upping your involvement in other more constructive activities if you notice that you're feeling like life is all 'goody-two-shoes' flat and dull. Choosing fresh activities that are inspirational as well as beneficial for the greater good helps to refresh and uplift the dynamic of your days.

Things I Would Love to Remember to Do Each Day...

I may not include every single one, every day, yet usually I do most of the list below. Your list of course will be customised by you, yet some of these may give you inspiration...

Tongue scraping
Neti pot
Drinking at least a gallon/4 litres of clean water
Yoga stretches/5 Tibetan Rites
Meditation for at least 15 minutes in the morning
Drawing an inspirational card from a pack
Skin brushing
Drinking fresh juice twice a day
Sweating
Bathing
Taking enzymes
Taking probiotics
Reading something inspirational
Giving something to another with no expectations
Cardio exercise that gets my heart beating faster
Spending time in nature
Breathing deeeeeeeep
Connecting in to the Universe repeatedly, through my whole chakra system
Greeting everything that graces my life with 'I love you', internally
Washing my feet before going to sleep
Connecting with friends socially
Sharing deep eye contact with someone I connect really well with
Speaking my truth in whatever context I am – staying centred
Experiencing nourishing physical contact with others

Where Do You Go From Here?

The exercises suggested in this book are simply *processes for your progress*: examining our patterns, questioning our histories, writing our Optimal Vision and so on. They aren't intended as places to get 'stuck'. Inquiring into these things is just part of the process to help you get to a more vibrant place. So be alert and take note if you seem to be getting bogged down along the way. Yes, it can feel very challenging when you start to examine your own emotional discord, yet opt for an overall positive outlook. Notice things as they come up for release; acknowledge them, *let them go*, move on. Rather than dwelling on any painful things that arise, maintain focus on where you **do** want to be – your highest vision for yourself. Keep moving forward, towards that vision of more vibrancy, joy and health. You now have many tools to create a more joyful, loving and healthy life for yourself. The choice is yours... What will you choose today...???

Your Emotional and Spiritual Recovery Checklist

This book has offered you an overview of the areas you might explore in emotional and spiritual recovery. In addition, the following Resources section contains many valuable extra pointers for you to investigate. After you've explored your own emotional/spiritual transformation for at least a few weeks, you might like to review the 20-point checklist that follows to monitor how you are feeling. Remember to be honest with yourself about where you really are right now and know that you are aiming for progress, not perfection. That you have read this far is the surest sign that you have what it takes to make sincere and lasting progress on this path of transformation. If ever you feel you have slipped off course, revisit this book and re-adjust your radar.

Every single moment is a point of fresh choice – and every fresh, positive choice is a seed of invigorating health and joy...

Do I...

- Identify my self-destructive behaviour and take action to develop new, healthy patterns?
- Acknowledge my defences, so that I have choices about using them less automatically?
- Identify my feelings in a healthy, assertive way, rather than eating over
- them?
- Develop trust in myself and others?
- Define my boundaries clearly?
- Choose not to 'wallow' in self-pity, blame and self-righteousness?
- Soften my all-or-nothing extreme thinking, choosing the middle ground instead?
- Say 'no' when I need/want/choose to? Say 'YES' to healthy choices, too?
- Spend time playing, having fun with friends and laughing? Regularly participate in welcoming company, rather than isolating myself?
- Find other ways to handle stress than overeating?
- Experience intimacy in my relationships with others?
- Cease co-dependent behaviour: stop trying to control/fix others or giving advice, explanations and apologies for being myself?
- Protect myself from destructive relationships, seeking outside help if necessary?
- Involve myself in group support work with others?
- Live with an 'attitude of gratitude' for life's gifts?
- Acknowledge a power greater than myself?
- Undertake regular prayer, meditation and reading of inspirational literature?
- Offer compassion and forgiveness to myself and others?
- Enjoy quiet and peaceful solitude rather than experiencing loneliness?
- Do my best to live now, in the moment?

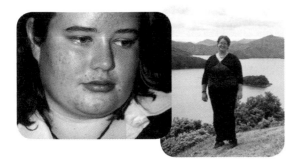

Then

If I can do it, I'm sure YOU can –
Blessings on Your Journey…

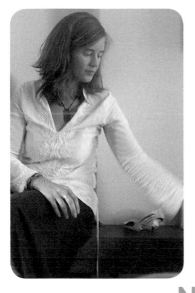

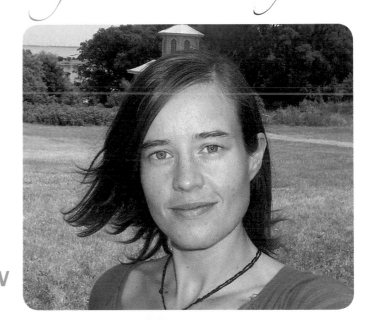

Now

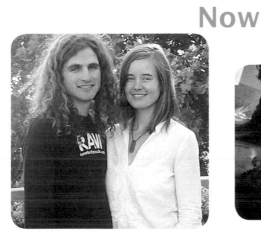

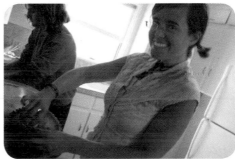

227

Appendix A: Twenty Tips for Healthy Raw Eating

This book is much less about *what* to eat as a raw foodist and more about what can happen beyond the physical when we *do* eat this way. However, I also want to provide here some brief, straightforward guidance for anyone who is a raw newbie and feeling confused about what to consume. Below you'll find twenty quick top tips (in no particular order) for shaping your own healthy raw lifestyle.

There are many ways to eat raw and the following is merely a simple set of guidelines that you *may* find useful. It is always wise to experiment for yourself and see what feels good to you. There are plenty of other resources out there to tap into for more information on these matters. For example, Matt Monarch's book *Raw Success* gives an excellent overview on how eating raw affects the physical body. My 30-Day raw weight loss programme is also designed to lead you step-by-step to a sustainable, healthy new lifestyle. You can learn all about that at www.RevitaLivePlan.com.

*Don't Eat Anything That Doesn't Rot

Processed foods, made with all kinds of preservatives and chemicals to prolong their 'shelf life', may take many years to break down, if ever. See shocking evidence of this on YouTube.com, where the 'Bionic Burger' video shows an intact collection of fast-food burgers dating back to 1989. These 'foods' haven't rotted, even after years. Imagine what things like this do inside your *body*.

*Choose Gluten-Free Foods

Wheat, rye, barley and oats – as well as spelt, couscous and kamut, to a lesser degree – all contain gluten. The protein gluten is a common food allergen; it clogs you up, slows digestion and is an intestinal irritant. Wheat flour mixed with water becomes *glue paste* – do you want to *eat* that...? Healthy alternatives include amaranth, buckwheat, corn/maize, rice, quinoa and millet, if you eat grains at all.

*Animal Products

It's not *necessary* to be vegan to benefit from being raw. People can feel genuinely healthy on animal products, *provided* they're raw – it's cooked/pasteurised animal foods that really cause a lot of damage. Eating cooked meat is like eating leather; it's very dense to digest. Pasteurised dairy is highly mucus-forming, acidifying and mineral-leaching. All 'ethics' aside, it's the *life force* of raw animal foods that can nourish people.

*Eat Whole Foods

Processed starches, refined sugars, trans-fats (manufactured, partially hydrogenated fats with long shelf lives, e.g. margarine) and so on cannot be easily recognised or used by the body. Aim for **whole foods** straight from the Earth instead (cooked if you like). Many vegetarians/vegans don't look so healthy, as they replace animal products with processed foods like pastas, bread etc. Remember: 'The middle aisles will kill you'!

*Vegetable Juice

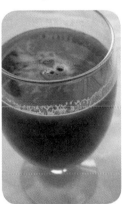

Drink veggie juice daily for optimal health. Use a range of vegetables, especially leafy greens. Veggie juice helps our body become more alkaline and offers incredibly fresh, highly absorbable nutrients. See Norman Walker's *Fresh Vegetable and Fruit Juices* book for more info. Drink at least one green veggie drink daily – preferably fresh juice – maybe a green smoothie, or even just green powder in water/coconut water.

*Mineral-Dense Foods

Most people are chronically demineralised, a result of both poor food choices and topsoil erosion. To balance out, consume lots of foods like seaweeds, seeds and nuts, chia, maca, dark green leafy vegetables, green powders, sprouts/greens grown with ocean water solution, etc. You can also supplement minerals if a blood/hair analysis shows a deficiency - take the angstrom or colloidal forms.

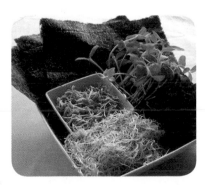

*Sprouts and Seaweeds

These are two major health keys for a modern raw foodist. Sprouts are packed with enzymes, are very easy and cheap to grow and give year-round fresh nourishment, anywhere. **Seaweeds** contain all the ocean minerals, including plenty of iodine, helping balance low thyroid activity. Nori and dulse are popular; I also love Sea Spaghetti and wakame. We sell many seaweed products in the RawReform Store.

*At Least 50% Raw

If *at least half* of what you eat is fresh raw food, you'll be on a **healing path**. That's 50% by the *weight* of the food and not the volume. (A salad weighs much less than pasta with meatballs, though they may cover half a plate each.) Of the raw foods you consume, also aim for at least 50% of those to be *fresh*/living raw foods, rather than dehydrated/packaged products.

*Food Combining

For digestive ease, eat simple combinations. Wild animals usually eat mono-meals. If we use five ingredients or fewer in meals, it's easier to digest. This can be refined over time. A few basic ideas: don't eat nuts and seeds, avocadoes, etc. (fats) with your fruits (sugars), or starchy veggies (e.g. yams) with *either*. Green leafy veggies combine well with everything. Keep melons separate from *all* other food.

*Blending

Some people find raw foods hard to digest; they may have weak stomach acid or not be used to much fibre. Sweet or savoury 'pre-digested' blended meals help, by breaking fibre down, making nutrient access easier. Few people chew well; blending food is like having the blender chew for you. Be sure to still chew smoothies in your mouth, though. Drinking celery juice daily is also great for raising up stomach acid.

*Be Cautious of 'Overlapping'

After consuming anything, leave time to finish digesting *that* before ingesting more. Otherwise, if you're still digesting some mango then eat a nut burger, you overlap digestive tasks and create issues. Ideally, eat fruit or drink veggie juice *before* a meal, on an empty stomach (for better absorption), then eat about thirty minutes later. Avoid fruit as dessert, or it gets stuck behind other foods and ferments.

*Avoid Eating Late at Night

Evening time is commonly recognised as the time of weakest digestion, in Chinese Medicine, Ayurveda, etc. Aim to stop eating at least three hours before you sleep, to give the body time to digest. Consider having your biggest meal of the day in the middle of the day. In terms of weight loss too, eating complex food combinations late at night makes releasing fat more challenging.

*Find Your Balance

Maintain a good *balance* of fruit, greens and fats in your intake, for optimal health. Fruits are 'aggressive' cleansers; eating lots of fruit can foster mood swings, anger, spaciness, ungroundedness etc., especially if you're not very active. Understand what you're doing to your body. Read Matt Monarch's book *Raw Success* (especially 'The Blood Gas Theory') for more on balance and detox.

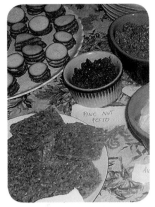

*Experimentation

Be open to trying new foods. If you've never tried barberries before, how will you know if you like them, or if your body 'needs' anything in them? Find satisfying new alternatives for *your* old favourites: e.g. cheese & crackers = dip & flax crackers now. Try out one or two new foods weekly. You may find that foods you didn't like before now taste nice to you, as your taste buds change.

*Detox Gently

If you're releasing fat, you're releasing toxins. You might feel weighed down/spacey/out of energy/depressed, etc., as toxins enter the bloodstream and potentially 're-tox' you. You can help your body move the waste out with colon cleansing, powdered enzymes, daily green juices and maybe even taking zeolites. Consuming **plenty** of greens helps the body balance, so it can release even those common 'stubborn last ten pounds'.

*Organic and Wild

Organic foods have a much higher nutrient and enzyme content. Using *non*-organic produce is actually *harmful* for you and the environment. Choose organic whenever possible, especially with water-rich produce like lettuce/celery/strawberries. Foraging your own wild food for free is a fabulous skill to develop. The vitality in fresh wild greens far exceeds shop-bought greens, even if they *are* organic.

*Supplements

Healthy raw foods and juices can be your 'medicine' now. There are also a few supplements you may find beneficial. Here are four I take regularly: probiotics to support my intestinal flora; enzymes to support every process of my body; kelp to support my thyroid; B-12 tablets as a 'back-up' in case my food/intestinal flora aren't providing plenty of this vitamin. All these products are available from the RawReform Store.

*Raw Food Travel
On trips, take heavier/dense/dried foods like nuts, seeds, flax crackers, goji berries, seaweed, chia seeds and so on. Then grab fresh produce and juices as and when you can. You might also want to travel with a little 'magic bullet' blender, to make dips/sauces/dressings. Travel with green powder, such as the product 'Greener Grasses'. It's always good to have green powders on hand, especially if you can't find fresh organic greens.

*Stimulants/Suppressants
It's rare to see raw foodists drink alcohol, coffee, black tea or colas/sodas. These items all sap the body's natural energy flow. Caffeine stimulates our adrenals, generating a false energy boost that ultimately drains us more. Alcohol places a huge strain on the whole body. Ceasing/minimising the use of these, along with other drugs – both recreational and prescribed – can greatly enhance health.

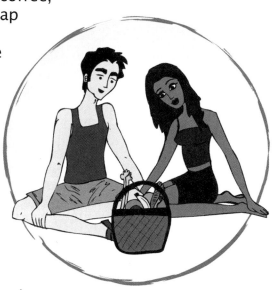

*Bless Your Food
The things you eat are about to literally 'become you' – try saying 'hello' first! If you pause before eating to bless your meal, give gratitude and visualise where it came from, this helps make the food less anonymous. It can also help you to centre, become present and relax, instead of 'diving in' to a meal, barely noticing the contents and eating quickly. Raise the vibration of your food with love and blessings.

Appendix B: Ten Easy Raw Recipes

Here are ten simple, practical recipes you can use to get started with a healthy raw lifestyle (if you haven't already). The recipes are all based on one person eating and have five ingredients or fewer, unless otherwise indicated.

'Chocolate Milk' Juice
½ a head of romaine lettuce
Bunch of spinach
6-8 medium-sized carrots

Run the veggies through your juicer and delight in the subtle similarity to chocolate milk.

Favourite Green Smoothie
2 bananas
1 juicy ripe mango
Big bunch of fresh spinach or other greens
Pure water

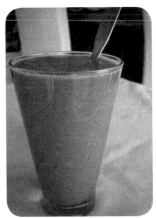

Separate out the mango flesh, throw all the ingredients in a high-speed blender with at least a cup of water (more if you like), blend and serve. Swap in other fruits and greens for variety.

Glass Jars
I recommend keeping aside a collection of glass jars of varying sizes, to store any leftover drinks, sauces, dips and so on. This is much better for your health than using plastic jars or pots, which may leach chemicals into your food.

Green Glow Soup
1 apple, cored
2 cups fresh greens – sunflower greens are delicious
Pure water
Chunk of ginger, peeled
Squeeze of lemon or lime to taste

Blend. Add some avocado for a 'fattier' soup.

Sunflower Pâté

1 cup soaked sunflower seeds
8-10 soaked sun-dried tomatoes
½ tbsp chopped garlic
Small bunch of basil

Mix all the ingredients together with a hand blender or food processor.

Simple Spaghetti

Big handful of kelp noodles OR sea spaghetti seaweed (soak sea spaghetti in water for at least an hour first)
1.5 tbsp nut or seed butter
Dash of apple cider vinegar or lemon juice to taste
Kelp granules/salty seasoning to taste
Pure water

Mix together the nut/seed butter with the water, kelp granules and vinegar into a thin dressing and pour over the noodles or sea-weed. Eat with joy! You can also blend in other flavours like garlic, fresh dill, basil and so on.

> **Kelp Noodles** are angel-hair noodle strands made from kelp seaweed. They contain only 18 calories per packet, are high in iodine, inexpensive and very easy to use, straight from the pack.
>
> **Sea Spaghetti** (Himanthalia elongata) is a delicious and nutritious seaweed, harvested mainly from the Atlantic Ocean. It looks just like spaghetti or linguini and once soaked, it has the texture of 'al dente' pasta.
> We sell kelp noodles, sea spaghetti and many other seaweeds, like nori and dulse, in the RawReform Store.

Seductively Squished Salad
(For 2)
Head of romaine lettuce sliced into thin strips OR a few handfuls of young salad greens
Small bunch of cilantro (coriander), chopped very finely
½ cucumber, grated
2 carrots, grated
½ red bell pepper, sliced into small chunks
Handful of dulse, shredded small
Juice of ½ lemon
Tsp kelp powder/salty seasoning to taste
Flesh of 1 avocado, in rough pieces

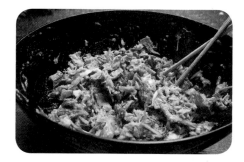

Any other 'garnishes' of choice – e.g. chopped chives, fresh sprouts, nuts

Combine all ingredients in a big bowl, then with your hand squish the whole mixture together until it's all evenly distributed and the avocado has spread out through the other ingredients, like a dressing. I believe the idea of squishing avocado through salad like this originated with Alissa Cohen. I love it because it removes the need for any other salad dressing (like heavy oils) and is so easy to prepare, with a minimum amount of fuss or equipment.

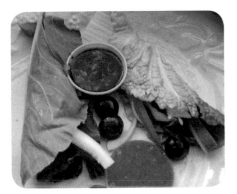

Romaine Roll-Ups

4-5 leaves of romaine lettuce per person
Assortment of grated/chopped vegetables
Favourite raw dips/sauces/spreads (e.g. the Sunflower Pâté above)
Dulse seaweed strips
Seeds and fresh herbs to garnish

Separate off big leaves from a head of romaine lettuce. Use the leaves as if they were tortilla wraps, filling them with the other vegetables, seaweed and dips, topping with seeds and herbs as desired. You can also use other large lettuce or cabbage leaves for roll-ups, along with nori sheets.

Sweet Shortbread Chia

4-5 tbsp chia seeds
2 cups fresh apple juice or blended apples
2 tbsp lucuma powder
¼ cup dried mulberries
¼ cup pumpkin seeds

Soak the chia seeds in the apple juice/sauce. Stir in the remaining ingredients. Leave to soak for at least 10 minutes before consuming.

Chia Seeds are tiny black and white, nutrient-dense seeds that swell up into a thick gel when soaked in liquid. They give a wonderful energy boost and are often referred to as the 'dieter's dream food'. You can read much more about chia on the RawReform Store website, where we sell the seeds, along with books on chia and a chia wall chart with recipes.

Lucuma Powder is a gorgeous shortbread-flavoured, low-glycemic sweetener. This yellowy-orange powder is made from a South American dried fruit and can be used in any sweet recipe. The Raw-Reform Store carries lucuma, along with other low-glycemic sweeteners such as mesquite and yacon powder.

Sweet Treats

(makes a big batch you can keep in the fridge)
1 cup of dried fruits of your choice, e.g. dates, figs, sultanas
2 big tbsp almond butter or other nut/seed butter
½ cup chopped nuts of your choice, e.g. walnuts, hazelnuts, pecans
2 tbsp raw carob or raw chocolate powder

Throw all ingredients into a food blender and mix until bound together in a big sticky lump. You might want to use a little water/liquid to help the blending. Divide out into small balls. You can create countless variations of this recipe – use different sweeteners like yacon syrup/powder or lucuma, for example. You could also add flavours such as orange, cinnamon and so on.

'Chocolate' Pudding

Flesh of one avocado
1 banana
1-2 tbsp raw carob or raw chocolate powder

Blend all the ingredients and enjoy. This can be adapted by adding in any flavouring, such as vanilla, thinning down to use as a sauce or thickening up with flax/chia seeds for a raw pie filling. You could sprinkle hemp seeds and bee pollen on top of this, to pack in more nutrients. (Incidentally, hemp seeds mixed with bee pollen is one of my favourite trail mixes to take on short trips.)

"Please, Miss, can I have some more...???"

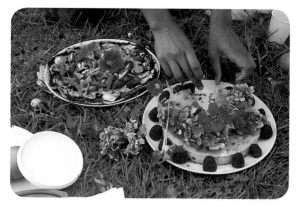

We sell many of the ingredients mentioned here in the RawReform Store, such as lucuma, dried mulberries, carob/chocolate powders, hemp seeds, chia seeds, dulse, nori, kelp noodles and sea spaghetti, as well as kitchen appliances like blenders, juicers and dehydrators.

For more raw recipe inspiration,

you can access our ongoing monthly meal planners as a 'Platinum' member of the Inner Circle community. See www.TheRawFoodWorld.com/ic for more information. I also recommend the websites GoneRaw.com and Living-Foods.com.

Personally, I very rarely use recipes anymore to make food – I just use what I have to hand and what seems like it would taste nice together. It can be very useful to have good reference books in the beginning though, so here's a list of ten of my favourite raw recipe books, in no particular order:

Ani's Raw Food Kitchen by Ani Phyo
Raw Living by Kate Magic
Shazzie's Detox Delights by Shazzie
Fresh by Valya and Sergei Boutenko
The Raw 50 by Carol Alt
Living on Live Food by Alissa Cohen
Raw Food Made Easy by Jennifer Cornbleet
Alive in 5 by Angela Elliott
Eating Without Heating by Valya and Sergei Boutenko
Raw Food for Busy People by Jordan Maerin

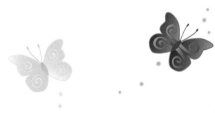

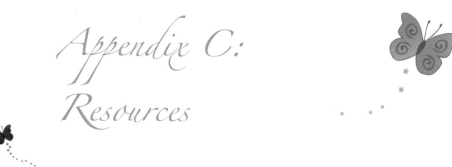

Appendix C: Resources

Please find contact details below for many of the items and techniques mentioned in this book. These resources are in no particular order.

RawReform Store

Among other things, we carry my e-books, the entire 'Anastasia' book series, *Non-Violent Communication* by Marshall Rosenburg, *The Law of Attraction* book, *The Secret* DVD and book, *Raw Success* by Matt Monarch, *Bliss Conscious Communication* by Happy Oasis, daily inspiration cards by Louise L. Hay, books on sprouting, raw recipe books and many of the other items mentioned in this text. You can visit the store at this website address: http://www.rawreform.com/store.

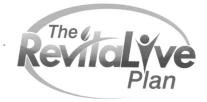

*RevitaLive Plan: http://www.revitaliveplan.com
My dynamic 30–day raw food weight loss programme. Enjoy our daily videos, meal planners, recipes, community support and fitness guidance.

*Inner Circle: http://www.therawfoodworld.com/ic
Our community site, the 'Inner Circle' (IC), where you can find support, access exclusive interviews and videos, chat, blog and more.

*The Raw Food World TV Show: http://www.therawfoodworld.tv
Our online TV show – regular videos of our raw adventures, recipes, interviews, travels, reviews and musings.

*Raw Success: http://www.rawsuccess.org
My partner Matt's site - there are many outstanding free articles and videos about raw food to enjoy.

*Spiritual Cinema: http://www.spiritualcinemacircle.com
Join this group to receive inspiring films sent straight to your house every month on DVD, to keep.

*Ho'oponopono: http://www.ancienthuna.com
Ho'oponopono is part of the simple yet powerful Hawaiian healing technique called Huna.

*Overeaters Anonymous: http://www.oa.org
The main site for OA.

*Co-dependents Anonymous: http://www.codependents.org
Find CoDA meetings.

*CWG: http://www.cwg.org
Main website for the Conversations With God Foundation.

*EFT: http://www.emofree.com
Emotional Freedom Technique – simple but extraordinary technique for healing. Download the free manual, read articles and more.

*Innertalk:http://www.innertalk.com
The full range of transformational subliminal CDs.

*Holographic Breathing: http://www.holographic-breathing.com Breathworker Buddhen's technique for body re-alignment using a unique breathing system.

*Cuddle Party: http://www.cuddleparty.com
Structured, safe cuddling workshops exploring boundaries, communication, intimacy and affection.

*David Deida: http://www.deida.info
Excellent resources about sacred intimacy, exploring masculine/feminine interaction.

*Caroline Myss: http://www.myss.com
Medical Intuitive, writer and speaker on energy healing, archetypes and spiritual practices.

*Retreats Online: http://www.retreatsonline.com
Worldwide directory of retreat centres.

*Four Season Farm: http://www.fourseasonfarm.com
Eliot Coleman's magnificent books on year-round organic vegetable farming, even in cold climates.

*Five Rhythms: http://www.gabrielleroth.com
Website of Gabrielle Roth, the originator of 'Five Rhythms' dancing/moving meditation.

*Living Alchemy: http://www.livingalchemy.co.uk
Jeanette McKenzie's amazing work using transformational perception shifts.

*Awakening With Horses: http://www.awakeningwithhorses.co.uk
Caro Des-Rivieres' powerful work linking horse communication and healing.

*Five Tibetan Rites: http://www.mkprojects.com/pf_TibetanRites.htm
For full details and illustrations of how to do these simple yoga moves.

*GITMR: http://www.giveittomeraw.com
Very supportive online raw food community - make your own profile, connect with others.

*Masaru Emoto: http://www.masaru-emoto.net
The groundbreaking work on the 'Hidden Messages in Water'.

*Philosopher's Notes: http://www.philosophersnotes.com/rawreform
Amazing collection of 'mini-CliffsNotes' for self-development books. Available in PDF and MP3 formats. Excellent free daily inspiring emails.

*Essene Gospel: http://www.essene.com/GospelOfPeace
Read the whole 'Gospel of Peace' for free on this site.

*Laughter Yoga: http://www.laughteryoga.org
Laugh your way to a healthier life!

*Dance of the Divine: http://www.danceofthedivine.org
Jacqui Lalita's glorious dance work helping women to release the goddess within.

*Non-Violent Communication: http://www.cnvc.org
A global organisation helping people connect compassion-
ately with themselves and one another.

*Hazelden: http://www.hazelden.org
World leaders in recovery work. Excellent resources, including free daily 'Gift for Today' emails.

*Permaculture: http://www.permaculture.org
A good starting point to find out more about 'permanent agriculture' methods.

*Global Ecovillage Network: http://gen.ecovillage.org
Central site for info on ecovillages and community living.

*Seeds of Change: http://www.seedsofchange.com
Outstanding collection of organic and heirloom seeds in N. America.

*Theta Healing: http://www.thetahealing.com
Learn all about theta and other brain waves from extraordinary healer Vianna
Stibl.

*Sprouting: http://www.sproutpeople.com
A gorgeous site for all things sproutable. See also Steve Meyerowitz's books
in the RawReform Store, along with our 'EasyGreen Sprouter' machines.

*SunFood Traveler: http://www.sunfoodtraveler.com
John McCabe's fabulous free global raw food resource list – raw restaurants,
books, sites, retreats and more.

*Scott Songs: http://www.scottsongs.com
The fabulously entertaining music of modern troubadour Scott Kalechstein.

*Story of Stuff: http://www.storyofstuff.com
Excellent twenty-minute, fast-paced, fact-filled film, exploring pro-
duction and consumption patterns in modern societies.

*Natural News: http://www.naturalnews.com
Mike Adams' outstanding site for cutting-edge news on alternative medicine and more.

*Positive News: http://www.positivenews.org.uk
Uplifting free newspaper published quarterly, covering 'positive news' world-wide.

*Post Secret: http://www.postsecret.com
Fascinating online project showing anonymous 'secrets', sent on postcards from people worldwide.

*TED: http://www.ted.com
An online collection of remarkable, inspiring talks, given by some of the world's foremost movers and shakers. Most of the talks are between three and eighteen minutes.

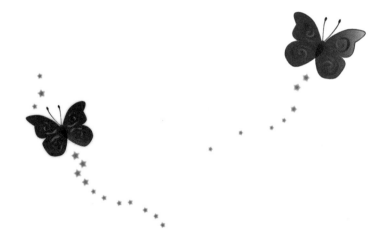

The RevitaLive Plan

– my 30-day raw food weight loss plan

I'm excited to offer this dynamic raw weight loss plan, including:

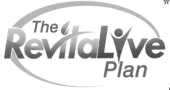

* daily instructional videos * meal planners * recipes (either all-raw or an 'Intermediate' plan with cooked options) * * community support * fitness guidance *

Learn all the practical tips that helped me release 160lbs of excess weight, maintain that weight loss and enjoy life more!

The daily videos deliver empowering tips you can start using immediately – it's like having me there in your home helping you! We cover how to:

★Release weight naturally using a system that has been proven.
★Let go of unsupportive habits that hold you back from your goals.
★Create simple, tasty meals and snacks for weight loss and health.
★Satisfy your sweet tooth and still stay healthy.
★Stick to your exercise plan.
★Find motivation ALL the time, whenever you want.
★Clear your mind from self-defeating chatter.

You can start this inexpensive 30-Day Plan at ANY time and we're so confident you'll love it that it even has a full money-back guarantee!

Here's what people have been saying about the RevitaLive Plan:

"I joined three days ago and am loving the plan!! Love the menus!
I'm noticing more **clarity** in my life and I feel more vibrant. I've lost 5 lbs in three days. Thank you thank you for the plan and for your example."
Traci

"Brilliant program. Love the videos...enjoying this immensely. Thank you!"
Lynn

"Thank you so much for this wonderful program. I've been eating raw for 5 days now and I already lost 10 pounds. Is that possible?! I cannot believe how fast it's going and how good I feel. I feel like a new person! wThis is coming from someone who has been a compulsive overeater all her life. I don't feel like I need to overeat anymore."
Alexandra

You can learn ALL about the RevitaLive Plan and join in the fun at
www.RevitaLivePlan.com. ENJOY!

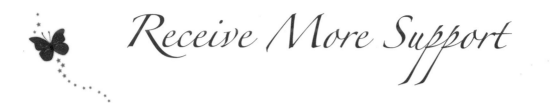

Receive More Support

Would you like my **personal** support on your journey of transformation?

I offer one-to-one **consultations**, as well as **group retreats**, for those exploring a raw lifestyle.

You can find out more by visiting the 'Consultations' page at the RawReform Store:

http://www.RawReform.com/store

Here's what others are saying about these consultations/retreats:

"Thank you for your help. I am down to 150 lbs and do I ever feel and LOOK GOOD! **Thanks for the advice – everything WORKS**!!! P.S., you should see how my skin has cleared up, and my hair is fuller, thicker, and it sure looks like there is more!!"
--RH, Ohio

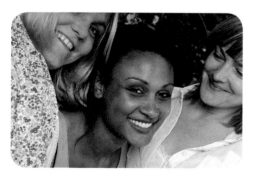

"Just wanted to say thank you for the consultation the other day; it was great! You were very informative and kind, and I'm really excited about taking this path. You look incredible in your pictures, and your story is amazing. I am very inspired by you; I know this is what I need also."
--AL, Pennsylvania

"I finally believe, at 47, and after so many years of addiction, that deep, true, lasting change is possible for me, on every level. I very much enjoyed speaking with you; I am just reviewing my notes, and reflecting on the many places your website has taken me. Thank you so much for all the inspiration."
Best,
--SW, Washington

"I want to tell you what a pleasure it was to work with you and your sensational program. You were more than amazing, you were a beacon to the women here that week-end. Letters and cards are pouring into the office. Thank you little 'Elfin-Fairy' for your vision, your journey in the RAW, your gentleness, kindness and class. You are loved by us all here."
--DJ at Ronora Lodge, Michigan

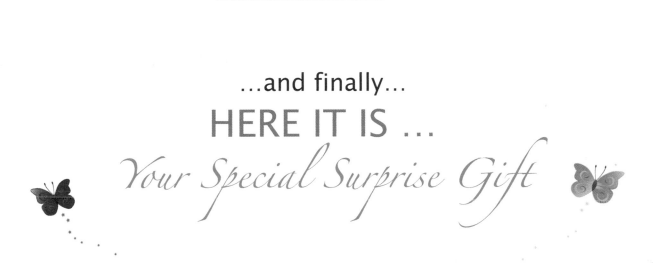

...and finally...

HERE IT IS ...

Your Special Surprise Gift

A whole collection of YUMMY, affirming, loved-up, sparkly slogans to take out and post up in YOUR vicinity, for happy little daily reminders of the wondrous being that you truly are...

(If you don't want to take this set of slogans out of your book, you can also go to the RawReform.com website and download these two pages from the 'Raw Emotions' area. You can then print the slogans out yourself, to decorate your space. Feel free to pass them on to others too – keep spreading the love!)

Turn to the next page and...

ENJOY!

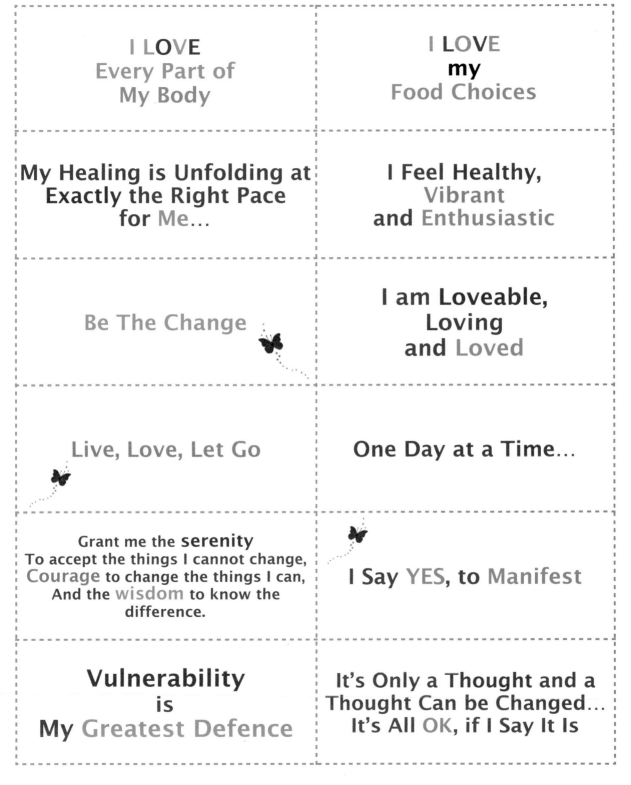

I LOVE
Every Part of
My Body

I LOVE
my
Food Choices

My Healing is Unfolding at
Exactly the Right Pace
for Me...

I Feel Healthy,
Vibrant
and Enthusiastic

Be The Change

I am Loveable,
Loving
and Loved

Live, Love, Let Go

One Day at a Time...

Grant me the **serenity**
To accept the things I cannot change,
Courage to change the things I can,
And the wisdom to know the
difference.

I Say YES, to Manifest

Vulnerability
is
My Greatest Defence

It's Only a Thought and a
Thought Can be Changed...
It's All OK, if I Say It Is

The Paths
are Many,
the Truth is One.

Thank You, I Love You,
Please Forgive Me,
I Am Sorry

I have
An Attitude
of Gratitude

Progress, not Perfection

I Am So Blessed

What Would LOVE Do Now?

Simplify,
Simplify,
Simplify…

The Only Constant
is
Change

I am
an
Active Transformer

I am Open
to Synchronicity, Flow, Joy
and Abundance

I choose beautifully

Joy is
my choice,
right now

Index